Hospital Acquired Infection and Legionnaires' Disease

Edited by Salim Surani and Joseph Varon

Published in London, United Kingdom

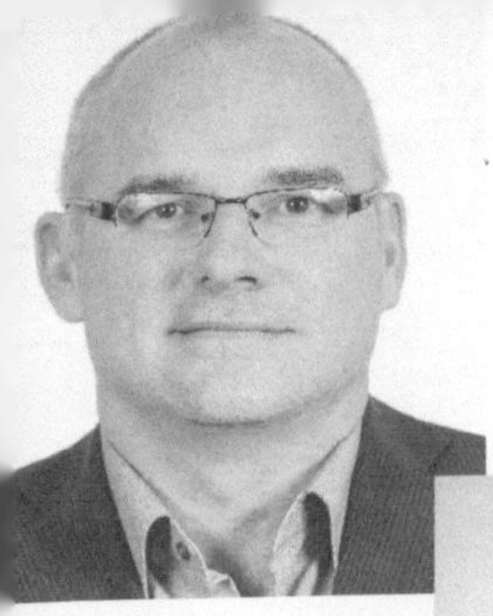
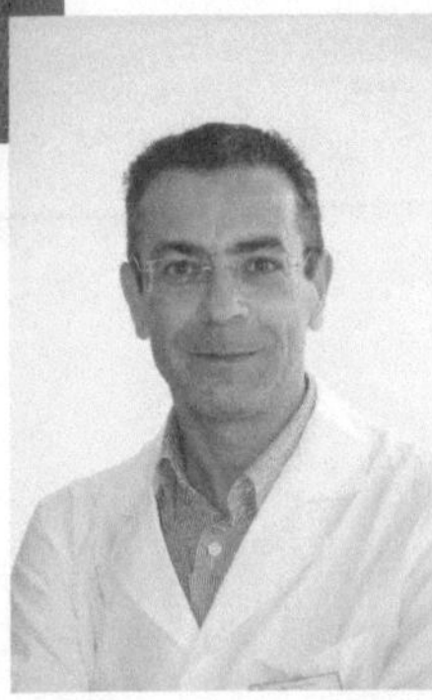
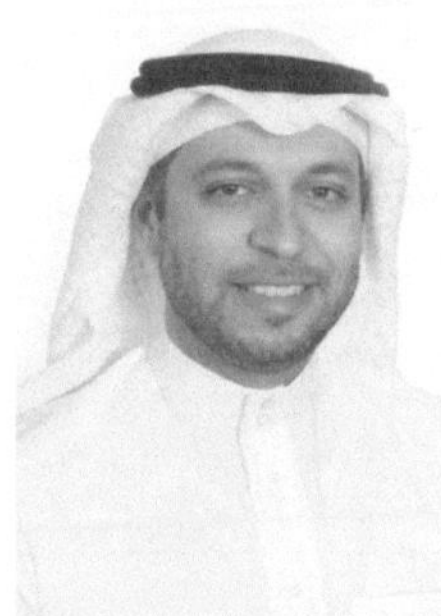
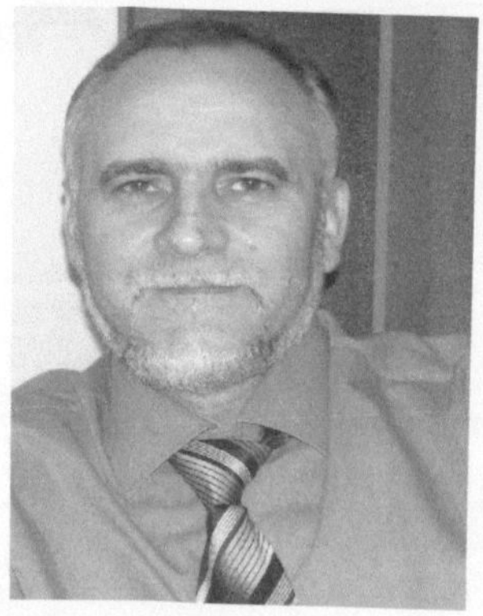
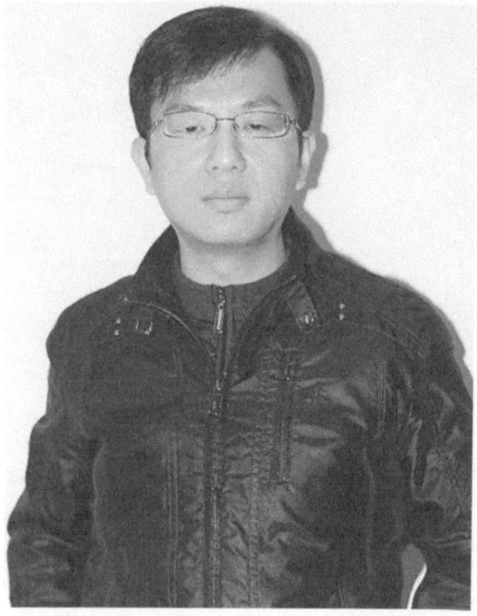
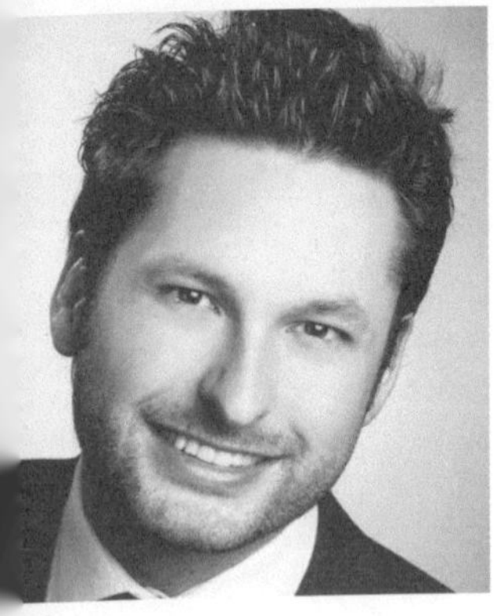
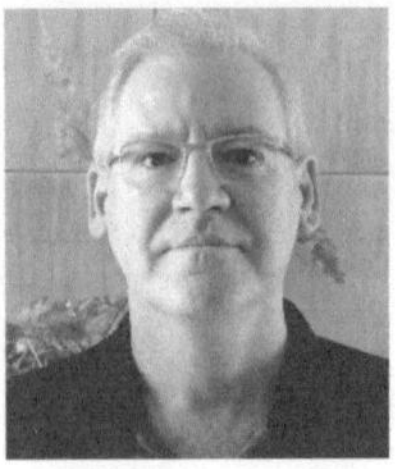

IntechOpen

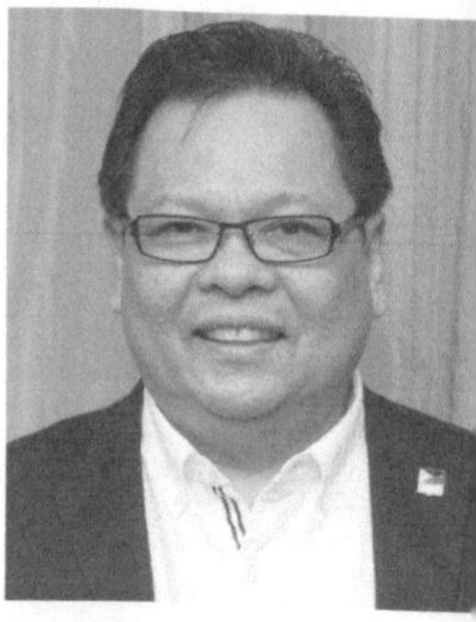
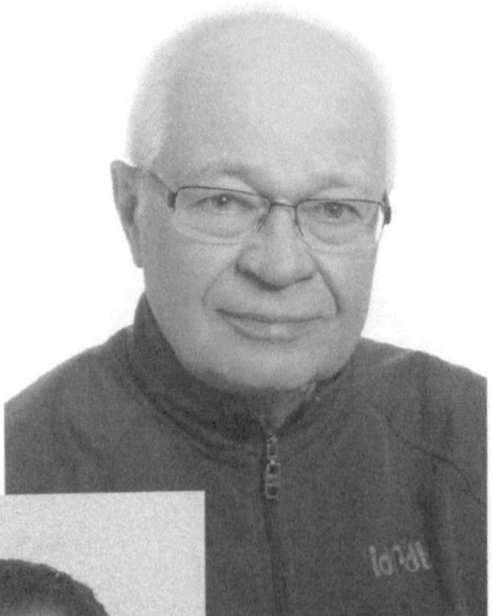
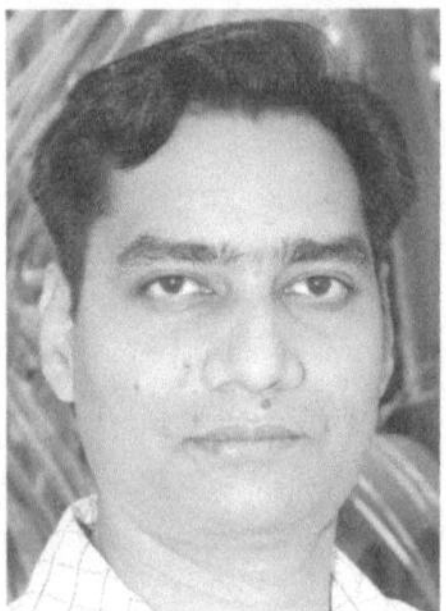
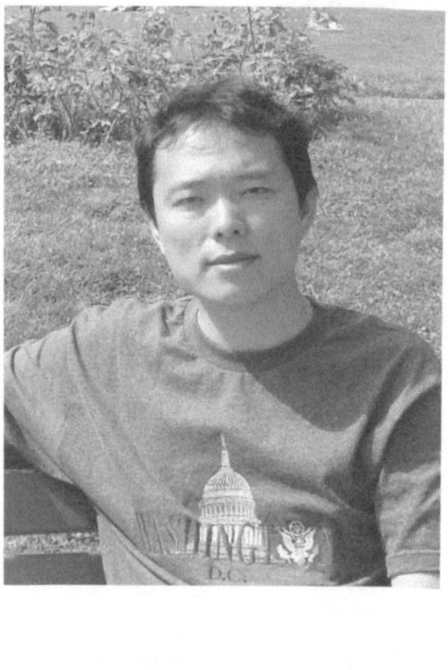
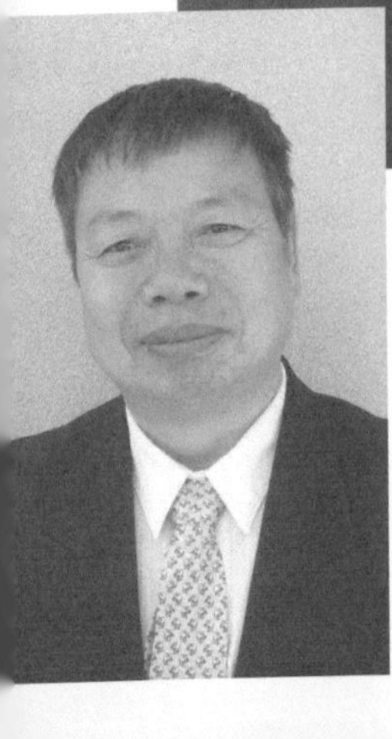
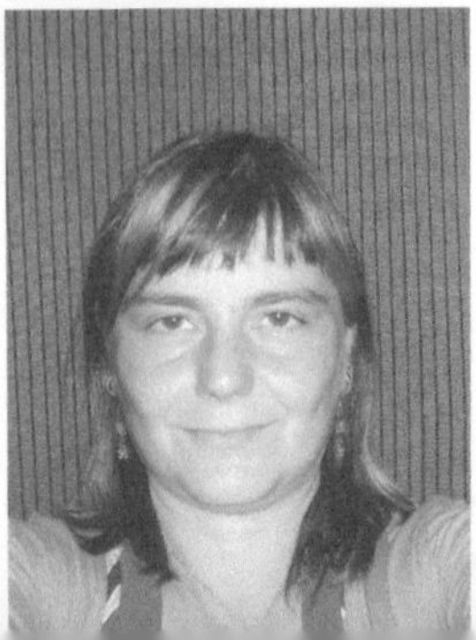

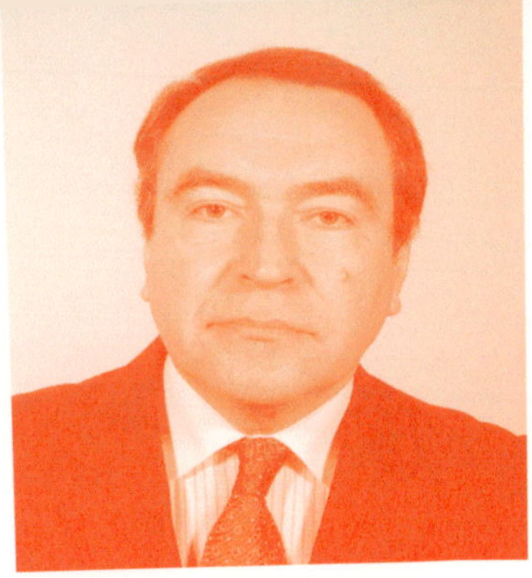
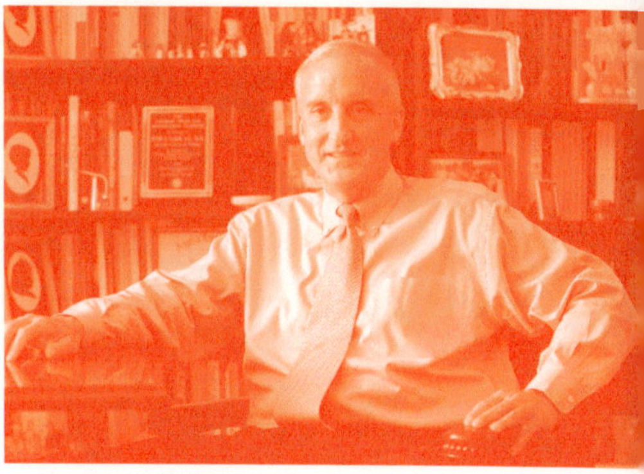
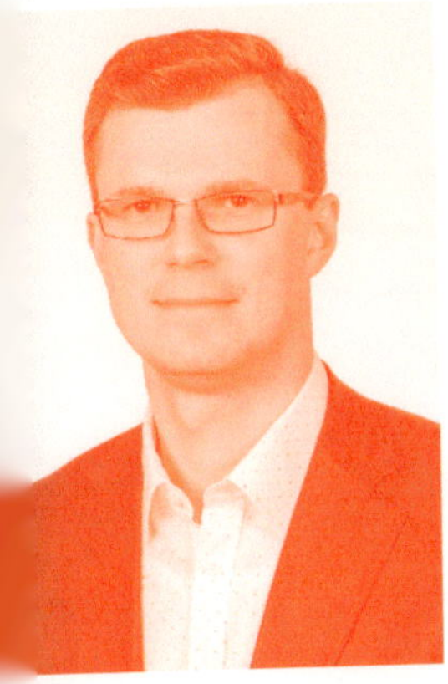
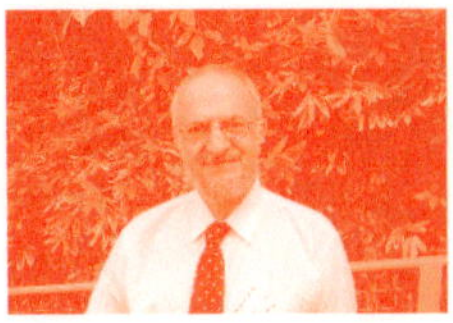
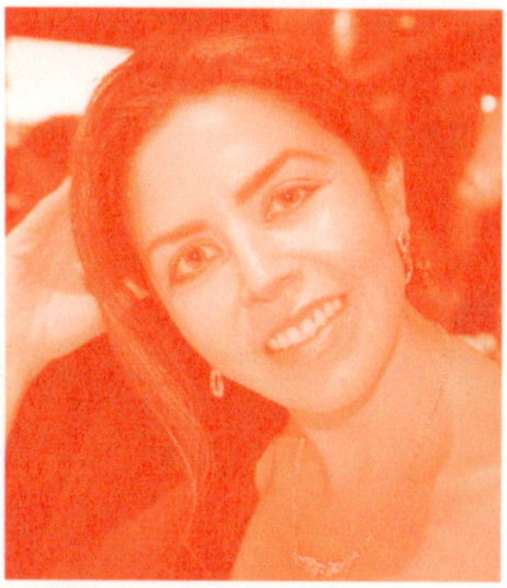

Supporting open minds since 2005

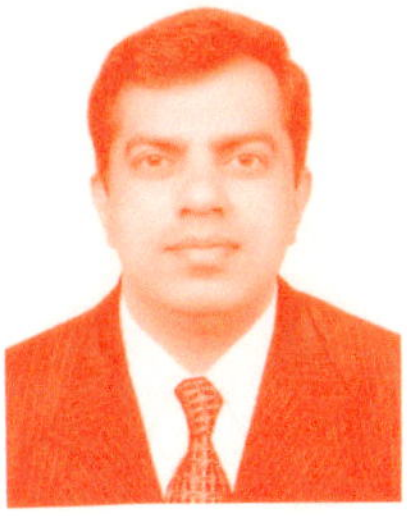
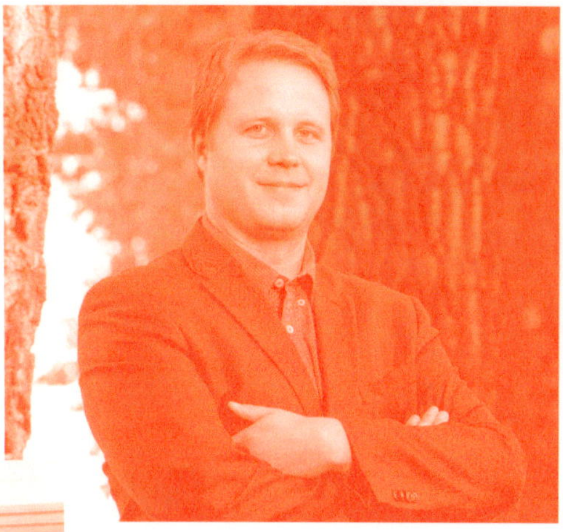
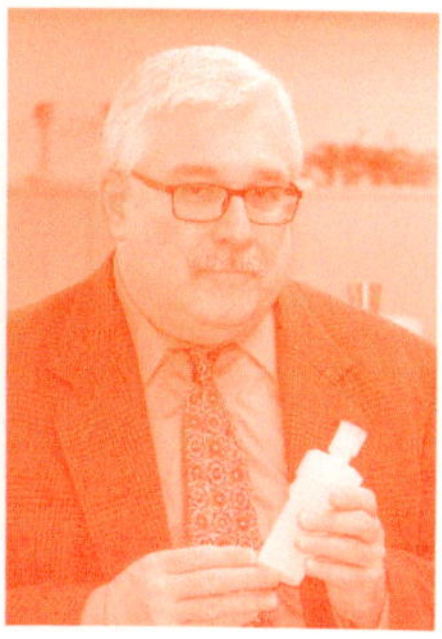
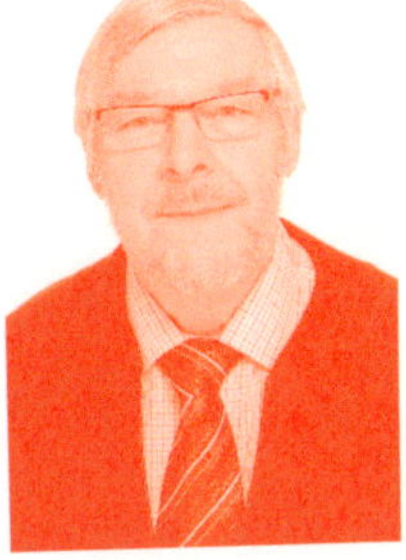
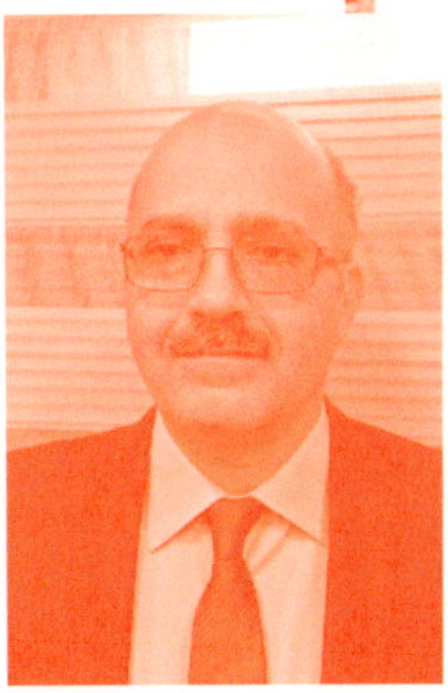
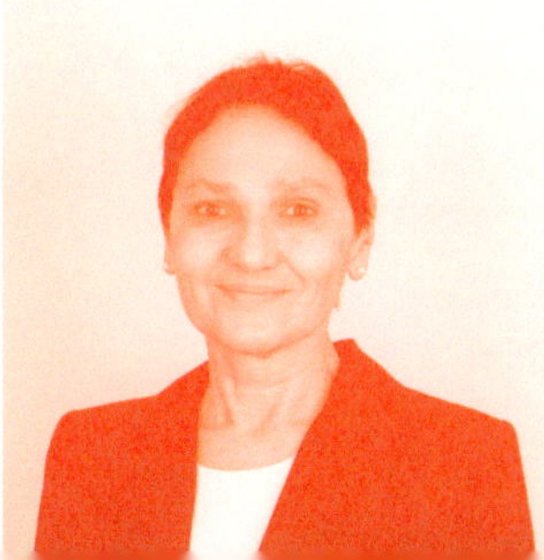
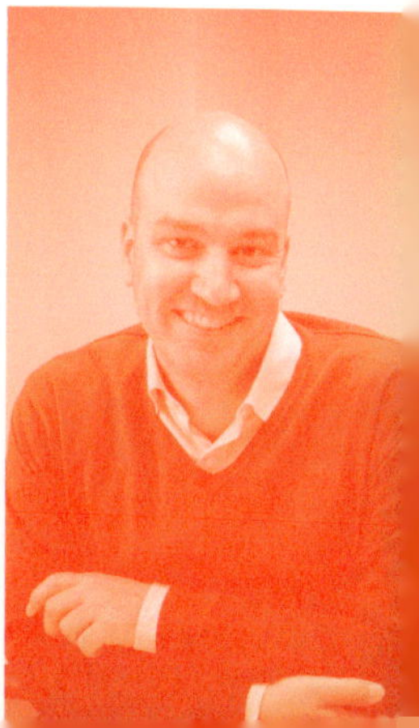

Hospital Acquired Infection and Legionnaires' Disease
http://dx.doi.org/10.5772/intechopen.83129
Edited by Salim Surani and Joseph Varon

Contributors
Jorge Velazco, Gilda Diaz-Fuentes, Ravish Singhal, Sindhaghatta Venkatram, Yamely Haydee Mendez, Ismael Garcia, Johanan Luna, Gloria Rueda, Venkat Rajasurya, Salim Surani, Akihiro Ito, Tadashi Ishida

First published in London, United Kingdom, 2020 by IntechOpen
IntechOpen is the global imprint of INTECHOPEN LIMITED, registered in England and Wales, registration number: 11086078, 7th floor, 10 Lower Thames Street, London, EC3R 6AF, United Kingdom
Printed in Croatia

British Library Cataloguing-in-Publication Data
A catalogue record for this book is available from the British Library

Additional hard and PDF copies can be obtained from orders@intechopen.com

Hospital Acquired Infection and Legionnaires' Disease
Edited by Salim Surani and Joseph Varon
p. cm.
Print ISBN 978-1-78985-969-0
Online ISBN 978-1-78985-970-6
eBook (PDF) ISBN 978-1-83880-300-1

Meet the editors

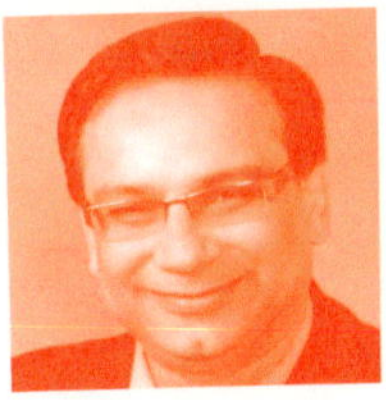

Dr. Salim R. Surani, MD, MPH, MSHM, FACP, FCCP, FAASM, currently works as the Chair of Critical Care Services at Corpus Christi Medical Center. He serves as Adjunct Clinical Professor of Medicine, Department of Pulmonary, Critical Care and Sleep Medicine at Texas A&M University. He also serves as the program director for the Pulmonary and Critical Care Fellowship Program at Bay Area Medical Center, Corpus Christi. He did his fellowship in Pulmonary Medicine at Baylor College of Medicine, Houston, Texas, his Masters in Public Health and Epidemiology at Yale University, and his Masters in Health Management at the University of Texas, Dallas. Dr. Surani has also served as board trustee and secretary of THE CHEST Foundation. He currently serves as co-chair for the ACCP Practice Operations Steering Committee. Dr. Surani has authored more than 150 articles in peer-reviewed journals and has written several books and book chapters. He has been involved in teaching residents for more than two decades. He was instrumental in starting an emergency medicine residency program, a pharmacy residency program, and a pulmonary and critical care residency program. He has been awarded Faculty of the Year Award numerous times. Dr. Surani has served as an independent grant reviewer for the government of Australia, as well as European nations via Rannis. He also serves as an ad hoc reviewer for more than 20 journals. He has served as a speaker in several regional, national, and international scientific conferences. His area of expertise includes critical care, sleep medicine, ICU infections, and practice operations. Dr. Surani serves on the Thursday morning health segment for Channel III news at Corpus Christi (ABC affiliate). He has also served on committees for several national organizations and has received several community and teaching awards, including the Health Care Hero award, and humanitarian awards for the American College of Physicians, American College of Chest Physicians, and Texas Medical Association. Dr. Surani is highly regarded among his peers and is well respected as a mentor, clinician, and humanitarian.

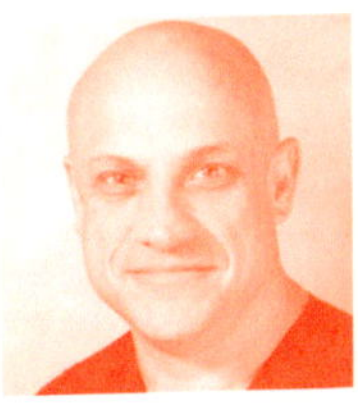

Dr. Joseph Varon is Professor of Acute and Continuing Care at the University of Texas Health Science Center in Houston, Texas, and was formerly Clinical Professor of Medicine at the University of Texas Medical Branch in Galveston. He is also Professor of Medicine, Surgery and Emergency Medicine at several universities in Mexico, the Middle East, and Europe. After completing medical training at the UNAM Medical School in Mexico City, Mexico, Dr. Varon served an internship in internal medicine at Providence Hospital, George Washington University, Washington, DC. A subsequent residency in internal medicine was completed at Stanford University School of Medicine in Stanford, California. Dr. Varon also served fellowships in critical care medicine and pulmonary diseases at Baylor College of Medicine in Houston. An avid researcher, Dr. Varon has contributed more than 790 peer-reviewed journal articles, 10 full textbooks, and 15 dozen book chapters to the medical literature. He is also a reviewer for multiple journals and currently serves as Editor-in-Chief for Critical Care and Shock and Current Respiratory Medicine Reviews. Dr. Varon has won many prestigious awards and is considered among one of the top physicians in the United States. He is also known for his groundbreaking contributions to critical care medicine in the fields of cardiopulmonary resuscitation and therapeutic hypothermia. He has developed and studied technology for selective brain cooling. He is also a well-known expert in the area of hypertensive crisis management. Along with Dr. Carlos Ayus, he co-described hyponatremia secondary to extreme exercise syndrome, also known as the "Varon–Ayus syndrome," and with Mr. James Boston he co-described the healthcare provider anxiety syndrome, also known as the "Boston–Varon syndrome." Dr. Varon has lectured in over 58 different countries around the globe. He has appeared in national and international television and radio shows with his techniques for the care of patients, along with Professor Luc Montagnier (Nobel Prize winner for Medicine in 2008).

Contents

Preface

Hospital acquired, or nosocomial, infections are very closely monitored for their prevention and control by regulatory agencies such as the Centers for Disease Control and Prevention and the US Department of Health and Human Services, with an emphasis on patient safety and quality of care. Currently, patient safety and quality of care have become key words. Critically ill patients in intensive care units are at higher risk of multidrug-resistant (MDR) infection. Excessive use of antibiotics, along with a host of multiple co-morbid conditions, predisposes patients not only to MDR infection but also to several atypical infections especially in the immunocompromised host.

Legionnaires' disease is a severe form of pneumonia caused by the bacteria *Legionella*. More than 10,000 patients are hospitalized every year with Legionnaires' disease in the United States alone. It is usually transmitted by inhaling the bacteria, commonly in the form of a mist. Those at risk are individuals with chronic lung conditions and the elderly and immunocompromised. The Legionnaire bacteria thrives in water. Contaminated water system(s) can be the source of infection by inhaling the aerosolized particles or aspiration of the contaminated water.

Legionnaires' disease is also an important public health topic as it involves environmental and public issues as far as spread and prevention are concerned. With an aging population, increasing number of transplants, increasing use of immunosuppressive medications, and compromised immunity due to multiorgan system disease, Legionnaires' disease is emerging as an important disease.

Moreover, extensive research and advances have been conducted in the areas of prevention, diagnostic modalities, and treatment. This book will try to address Legionnaires' disease in the hospital setting, in addition to MDR infection.

Salim Surani, MD, MPH, MSc, FACP, FCCP, FAASM
Adj. Clinical Professor of Medicine,
Texas A&M University,
Health Science Center,
College of Medicine,
Texas, USA

Section 1

Introduction

Chapter 1

Introductory Chapter: Hospital-Acquired Infection and Legionnaires' Disease

Salim Surani

1. Introduction

According to the Institute of Medicine, hospital-acquired infection and the adverse event in hospitals are responsible for 44,000–98,000 deaths and account for $17–29 billion in the healthcare cost in the USA alone [1, 2]. The care of the patient in the intensive care unit (ICU) is expensive and poses a significant economic burden on the healthcare [3, 4]. In the early part of the twentieth century, the intensive care units were taking care of patients with respiratory failure related to polio. With the advancement of technology and medicine, patients with multiple comorbidities are now being admitted in the ICU. A study by the World Health Organization (WHO) found that 51% of the patients in the ICU have infections [5]. The risk of infection among patients on a mechanical ventilation is 6- to 21-fold higher. Surprisingly, the risk of ICU-acquired infections among low- and middle-income countries was found to be 2–3 times higher than the ICU-acquired infections among ICU patients in developed countries [5, 6]. With the advent of invasive monitoring and therapeutic devices, the incidence and prevalence of the infection have increased, and we have seen a significant increase in antibiotic use and multidrug-resistant (MDR) infections [7]. Infectious conditions, sepsis, and septic shock continue to be responsible for significant morbidity and mortality [7]. Increased MDR infection has now become a global threat. Two million cases and 23,000 deaths each year are attributable to MDR infection in the USA alone, according to the Centers for Disease Control and Prevention (CDC) [8, 9]. In addition, inappropriate use of the antibiotics not only leads to increase in MDR but costs the healthcare $27–42 billion annually [8–10]. The central line-associated bloodstream infection (CLABSI) and catheter-associated urinary tract infection (CAUTI) have also been associated with significant nosocomial infection [11]. With significant efforts from the regulatory agency as well as the healthcare organization and providers, a significant decrease in CLABSI and CAUTI has been seen [1, 12]. Education and antibiotic stewardship programs have been recommended by the CDC in 2014. In 2017, a survey by the National Healthcare Safety Network found that the number of hospitals with antibiotic stewardship program (ASP) has increased to 76.4%. Still 25% of the hospitals do not have ASP. As of September 2019, the ASP is required by the Centers for Medicare and Medicaid Services (CMS) as part of the patient care reimbursement. With this new regulatory requirement by the CMS, it is expected that the ASP in hospitals will reach close to 100% [13].

In this book, we will also be addressing Legionnaires' disease in detail. Legionnaires' disease is a bacterial infection caused by Gram-negative bacteria, usually found in freshwater [14]. It can lead to severe pneumonia which can be fatal

Country	City/state	Source	Cases	Mortality	Fatality rate
London, England [17]	Westminster	Via. water system	3	0	0
Belgium [18]	Evergem	Cooling towers	32	2	6.7%
USA [18]	Ohio, New Jersey, Michigan	Unknown? Flint Michigan water crisis	32	6	18.75%
USA [18]	Atlanta, Georgia (in Sheraton Hotel)	Water system	66	1	1.5%
USA [18]	Fletcher, North Carolina	Hot tub display	141	4	2.83
Canada [18]	Moncton, New Brunswick	Unknown	16	N/A	—
USA [18]	Batavia, Illinois		13	N/A	—

Table 1.
Selected Legionnaires' disease outbreak in 2019.

(Legionnaires' disease), but milder and subclinical infection forms (Pontiac fever) do exist [14, 15]. This disease is much more common than we think. Approximately, 10,000 patients are hospitalized every year with Legionnaires' disease in the USA alone. Legionnaires' disease also creates a public health concern. It is usually transmitted by inhaling the mist or via the cooling and water system issues. There have been numerous Legionnaires' disease outbreaks over the decades, and the number seems to be increasing [16]. In the 1970s there were five outbreaks, in the 1980s seven, in the 1990s four, and in the 2000s ten. From 2010 to 2018, there were 23 outbreaks. In the year 2019 alone, there were seven outbreaks (shown in **Table 1**). These reported outbreaks represent just the tip of the iceberg, as not all of them are reported. Moreover, reports from the developing countries are almost nonexistent. The fatalities from Legionnaires' disease range from 0 to 75% [16]. The longevity, multiple invasive devices, increase in transplants, immunocompromised status, aging population, and increase in travels all pose a significant risk of increased outbreaks and high fatality rates. Research and education need to be done in this area. In this book, we will try to address the epidemiology, clinical and therapeutic as it pertains to disease as well as clinical scenario and treatment of Legionnaires' disease among immunocompromised host.

Author details

Salim Surani
Health Science Center, College of Medicine, Texas A&M University, Texas, United States

*Address all correspondence to: srsurani@hotmail.com

References

[1] Eggimann P, Pittet D. Infection control in the ICU. Chest. 2001;**120**(6): 2059-2093

[2] Brennan TA, Leape LL, Laird NM, Hebert L, Localio AR, Lawthers AG, et al. Incidence of adverse events and negligence in hospitalized patients. Results of the Harvard Medical Practice Study I. The New England Journal of Medicine. 1991;**324**(6):370-376

[3] Garland A, Olafson K, Ramsey CD, Yogendran M, Fransoo R. Epidemiology of critically ill patients in intensive care units: A population-based observational study. Critical Care (London, England). 2013;**17**(5):R212

[4] Murthy S, Adhikari NK. Global health care of the critically ill in low-resource settings. Annals of the American Thoracic Society. 2013;**10**(5): 509-513

[5] Organization WH. Healthcare Associated Infections Fact Sheet. 2016. Available from: http://www.who.int/gpsc/country_work/gpsc_ccisc_fact_sheet_en.pdf

[6] Iwuafor AA, Ogunsola FT, Oladele RO, Oduyebo OO, Desalu I, Egwuatu CC, et al. Incidence, clinical outcome and risk factors of intensive care unit infections in the Lagos University Teaching Hospital (LUTH), Lagos, Nigeria. PLoS One. 2016;**11**(10):e0165242

[7] Hranjec T, Sawyer RG. Management of infections in critically ill patients. Surgical Infections. 2014;**15**(5):474-478

[8] Ventola CL. The antibiotic resistance crisis: Part 1: Causes and threats. P & T: A Peer-reviewed Journal for Formulary Management. 2015;**40**(4):277-283

[9] Ventola CL. The antibiotic resistance crisis: Part 2: Management strategies and new agents. P & T: A Peer-reviewed Journal for Formulary Management. 2015;**40**(5):344-352

[10] Ventola CL. Evaluation of Biosimilars for formulary inclusion: Factors for consideration by P&T committees. P & T: A Peer-reviewed Journal for Formulary Management. 2015;**40**(10):680-689

[11] Angus DC, Pereira CA, Silva E. Epidemiology of severe sepsis around the world. Endocrine, Metabolic & Immune Disorders Drug Targets. 2006;**6**(2):207-212

[12] Eggimann P, Hugonnet S, Sax H, Harbarth S, Chevrolet JC, Pittet D. Long-term reduction of vascular access-associated bloodstream infection. Annals of Internal Medicine. 2005;**142**(10):875-876

[13] Policy Cfidra. New Rule Requires Antibiotic Stewardship Programs in US Hospitals. University of Minnesota; 2019. Available from: http://www.cidrap.umn.edu/news-perspective/2019/09/new-rule-requires-antibiotic-stewardship-programs-us-hospitals

[14] Fields BS, Benson RF, Besser RE. Legionella and Legionnaires' disease: 25 years of investigation. Clinical Microbiology Reviews. 2002;**15**(3):506-526

[15] Glick TH, Gregg MB, Berman B, Mallison G, Rhodes WW Jr, Kassanoff I. Pontiac fever. An epidemic of unknown etiology in a health department: I. Clinical and epidemiologic aspects. American Journal of Epidemiology. 1978;**107**(2):149-160

[16] List of Legionnaires' disease outbreaks: Wikipedia; 2020. Available from: https://en.wikipedia.org/wiki/List_of_Legionnaires%27_disease_outbreaks

[17] Health officials probe case of deadly Legionnaires' Disease at one of London's most famous apartment blocks: Evening Standard. 2019. Available from: https://www.standard.co.uk/news/london/health-officials-probe-case-of-deadly-legionnaires-disease-at-one-of-londons-most-famous-apartment-a4096926.html

[18] Support LaaMP. 2019. Available from: https://hcinfo.com/about/outbreaks/recent/

Section 2

Epidemiology

Chapter 2

A Clinical Overview of Hospital-Acquired Legionella Pneumonia: Prevention Is the Key?

Yamely Mendez, Gloria Rueda, Ismael Garcia and Johanan Luna

Abstract

Legionella pneumophila is a Gram-negative bacteria that cause community-acquired pneumonia in very common circumstances. Although it is rare to develop hospital-acquired pneumonia due to *Legionella pneumophila*, there are cases where the infection appears during its presence in the hospital environment or because of the existence of Legionella outbreaks. It is important to mention that the colonization of this organism is mostly found in some hospital water supplies. The prevention of the spreading of this nosocomial pathogen is crucial for the hospital setting by identification of the bacteria. Using surveillance and control of infection, as well as maintaining beneficial isolation of those patients with the disease, could prevent the dissemination of this rare infection among hospitalized patients that are highly vulnerable. The treatment should be effective and according to the standard of care guidelines. The initiation of empiric antibiotic therapy is critical once the pathogen is suspected to be the etiology of pneumonia.

Keywords: legionella pneumonia, hospital, hospital-acquired, prevention, clinic, epidemiology, pneumonia, management

1. Introduction

Legionnaires' disease is a severe type of pneumonia. It is typically acquired by inhalation of contaminated water containing the *Legionella pneumophila* gram-negative bacteria. The severe pneumonia occurs most frequently in susceptible patients (i.e., former or current smokers, chronic diseased patients, immunosuppressed patients and those >50 years of age) [1]. The most commonly transmission of contaminated water is from showerheads, some medical equipment (i.e., respiratory devices), cooling towers, hot tubs, hydrotherapy equipment's and/or decorative water fountains [2]. Several countries have different recommended strategies for the prevention of *Legionella pneumophila* dissemination. They measure dangerous concentrations and they use water sampling frequency with activation of alerts of the *L. pneumophila* levels. These strategies always depend on local regulations and the geographic variations. Although, the regulations have some differences, all of them include three principles: (1) the supervision of critical spots (which are locations in a hot water installation where water stays, and makes the *L. pneumophila* in a suitable growth temperature range for some time), (2) avoiding water stagnation in specific parts of the system and the prevention of the proliferation and (3) requirement of a sufficiently high temperature to prevent the growth and spread of *L. pneumophila*. The European Working Group for Legionella Infections recommends that the total volume of the storage tank needs to be heated to 60°C for at least an hour a day, depending on the risk of spreading [3]. In the United Kingdom, the Department of Health recommends maintaining hot water temperatures at a temperature lever >55°C and cold water <20°C to prevent the proliferation of *L. pneumophila* in the water systems. Also, when cooper and silver ionization is introduced to a new building in conjunction with appropriately managed water, there is a better control in the dissemination of the bacteria [4]. It is important to mention that Legionella prevention should start with the correct design and construction of the water networks. During facilities renovations or a construction of a new one, the pipe runs should be as short as practical [5]. Usually, the evaluation of water systems for Legionella is until after the disease has been identified and confirmed. Thus, it is recommended a practical approach of periodic testing for Legionella, along with proper water treatment to avoid large-scale outbreaks [6]. In addition of water management in all health care facilities, it is crucial to have better methods for detecting Legionella in the water systems and in some of the clinical specimens to enhance the preventive strategies and the clinical diagnosis. In the United States, the CDC developed a toolkit to for all Medicare-certified healthcare facilities to assist in the water management in order to reduce the growth and transmission of the bacteria [7].

One of the preventive methods is to run cultures and other diagnostic methods to assess the rate of spreading of the gram-negative bacteria. According to a study made in Pittsburgh, Pennsylvania, water cultures are more significantly more sensitive than collected swab cultures in detecting *Legionella pneumophila*. This study was done due to an outbreak of nosocomial Legionnaires' disease among 22 veterans in the Veterans Affairs Pittsburgh Healthcare System [8]. The reality is that testing for atypical pathogens in patients is poorly standardized in a realistic scenario, especially in low-income countries where some guidelines are needed for the implementation of a suitable diagnosis. One of the major implications of this approach is the wide heterogeneity across continents and countries [9].

The risk management in hospitals of *Legionella pneumophila* seems to be underrepresented in the literature. A literature review done by Leiblein, et al., stated that further research in the field of risk management and prevention of Legionella in the water systems must be perform [10].

2. Epidemiology

All Legionnaires' disease cases are reported to the Centers for Disease Control and Prevention (CDC). In 2015, a national surveillance data confirmed a total of 2809 Legionnaires' disease cases. Those cases were reported to the CDC from 21 jurisdictions, including 85 definite (3%) and 21 (17%) possible health-care associated cases. This last high rate marks the importance of case prevention among health institutions and the implementation of effective water maintenance programs, as well as a proper case identification. The most frequent health-care facility associated with this disease was a long-term care facility, with 80% of the definite cases [11]. In the United States, the reported cases of Legionnaires' disease have increased nearly 4.5 times since the year 2000. It could be related to the increased susceptibility of the population, the access to new diagnostic methods or a combination of both [12]. One of the main causes of transmission is closely related to professions where there is nebulization with water, mainly among workers with long term exposure. The outbreaks tend to be seasonally, especially in the hottest months of the year (May–August) [13].

Although, it is historically associated with healthcare institutions, it is important to mention that some retirement homes are also at risk of dissemination of the disease. The healthcare-associated cases represent a proportion of cases in elderly patients (>60 years of age). Drinking contaminated water can contribute to outbreaks. De Filippis, et al., collected hot water and biofilm samples from showerheads of retirement homes. Then they were tested by culture method. It resulted in 140 hot water and biofilm samples collected, with Legionella found in 36.8% of the samples. The results suggested that the colonization of these retirement homes is occasional, but further studies were suggested [14].

Although there are limited data available, the incidence reported is around 10–15 cases detected per million population. From them, 75–80% are >50 years and 60–70% are male with underlying chronic diseases [15].

Nevertheless, the prevention of Legionella still remains a critical issue, even in healthcare facilities where monochloramine disinfection has been introduced. It is documented that monochloramine has a better impact that free chlorine alone on Legionella control [16].

Although, this makes that continuous treatments with low monochloramine doses induced a viable but non-culturable state of Legionella. A study made by Casini, et al., obtained water and biofilm samples and isolated Legionella with the use of standard procedures. It emphasized the importance of keeping an appropriate and uninterrupted monochloramine dosage to ensure the control of *L. pneumophila* colonization in water supplies for hospitals [17].

Another chemical disinfection method used in water systems is the chlorine dioxide. It is reported that the duration of the effective protection of chlorine dioxide is reliable and could support the process in the framework of risk management activities in hospitals. This was documented by Vincenti, et al., where the duration of chlorine dioxide method in eradicating Legionella was analyzed in a large hospital in Rome. The observation was made from samples takes between 2011 and 2018. It concluded that Legionella was never detected at 4 years of follow-up [18].

3. Pathophysiology

Legionella pneumophila can be found in biofilm formations, as a single microbe in freshwater and manmade devices such as, shower heads, air conditioning systems, cooling towers and water fountains. This intracellular pathogen is the causative agent of a severe form of pneumonia known as legionnaires' disease [19]. Once transmission to the human lung is established through inhaled infectious aerosols, *L. pneumophila* is engulfed by the macrophage where it replicates, causes inflammation and consequently pneumonia [20]. Jäger et al., showed, through human lung tissue explants that *Legionella pneumophila* damage to lung is characterized by "destruction of its connective tissue, proteinaceous exudate and delamination of alveoli", [21] thus the physical symptoms.

L. pneumophila obtains shelter from harsh environmental conditions by forming an advantageous relationship with unicellular protozoa. Besides shelter it provides nutrients for survival and infectivity. Once *L. pneumophila* utilizes all the protozoa's nutrients, it exits the host as bacterium capable of thriving within monocytes and macrophages in case of inhalation through the infected particles. Once inhaled, the bacteria reach the alveoli, enter alveolar macrophage through coiling phagocytosis or normal phagocytosis, and cause legionnaires' disease. Previous studies have shown that this is thanks to genes that encode for effector proteins with eukaryotic characteristics that are injected through the legionella containing vacuole. This is known as molecular mimicry [19, 22]. Cazalet et al., found 30 genes of *L. pneumophila* that encoded for proteins with high resemblance to eukaryotic proteins and another 32 genes involved in protein-protein interactions within eukaryotic domains [23].

3.1 Strategy

Legionella's life cycle consists of two main phases. In order to survive against harsh environmental conditions, legionella enters a "reversible dormant state", known as the viable but not culturable state (VBNCS) [24]. When environmental conditions improve, like in the case of phagocytosis by *Acanthamoeba castellanii*, the bacterium represses its virulent traits and goes into its exponential phase, in which it replicates within the protozoa [6]. This process of replication takes round 15 hours to complete [25]. Once lack of nutrients and environmental stress strikes, *L. pneumophila* coordinates its differentiation to the mature intracellular form (MIF) and the stationary phase form (SPFs), both with virulent traits characterized by high motility and cytotoxicity and proceeds to lyse the cell and infect cells in proximity. Although studies are lacking on the mechanisms by which the host cell is lysed by the bacterium [24, 25]. SPFs present flagella, loose outer membrane, and a well-defined inner membrane, while MIFs typically appear as stubby rods with complex envelope, both being able to colonize alveolar macrophages [24]. Legionella accomplishes this physiologic and morphologic change by the coordination of LetA/LetS and sigma factors RpoS and FiA [26]. When there is low availability of amino acids, RelA, a ribosomal enzyme, synthetizes alarmone ppGpp (guanosine pentaphosphate) with subsequent activation of sigma factor RpoS and LetA/S. LetA/S work in conjugate to induce the expression of CsrB homologues which are RNAs that can sequester CsrA. CsrA expression represses the flagellar sigma factor fliA, which translates into a non-motile pathogen, with reduced virulence [27]. Studies have shown that through legionella's exponential phase, the bacterium increases its resistance against heat, and antibiotics [24].

3.2 Legionella and the host cell

The key mechanism for *L. pneumophila* inert ability to survive against the harsh intracellular environment is its secretory system. *Legionella pneumophila* uses a type IVB secretion system (T4BSS) encoded by the delayed in organ trafficking/intracellular multiplication gene [28]. The T4BSS is involved in endocytic and secretory pathways as well as ubiquitination, host lipid metabolic exploit and cell death prevention by enabling the formation of the vacuole in which the bacterium resides for multiplication [29]. When a phagosome is formed, it matures, acidifies, and fuses with the lysosome. The phagolysosome can digest the contained organism through different bactericidal peptides, reactive oxygen species (ROS) and hydrolytic enzymes. Once the pH of the phagolysosome achieves certain acidity, these hydrolytic enzymes get activated leading to the destruction of the pathogen [28]. The acidification is accomplished by a proton pump ran by ATP hydrolysis called the vacuolar-ATPase (v-ATPase). This v-ATPase is made up by the trans-membrane domain V_0, and the cytosolic V_1 domain, which translocate H^+ across the lipid bilayer and hydrolyzes ATP used for proton translocation respectively [30]. Prior research suggests that *Legionella pneumophila* secretes SidK, an effector protein that halts acidification of the phagolysosome by interaction with v-ATPase in early stages of infection. Zhao et al. showed that Binding of Sidk to the v-ATPase decreased its affinity, although only by 40% of v-ATPase activity, suggesting the presence of other effector proteins [30].

A key element on the formation of the LCV is the ability to disrupt vesicle trafficking between the ER and the Golgi apparatus. This interception of vesicle is what gives the LCV the ability to expand for replication and its ER-like properties [31].

Multiple studies show that *L. pneumophila* can accomplish this by targeting Rab1, a member of the Ras superfamily GTPases. Rab proteins are essential to the secretory pathway, and these proteins are localized in specific intracellular membranes, mainly ER and Golgi [32]. Control over inactive GDP-bound and active GTP bound GTPases are controlled by Guanine nucleotide exchange factors (GEFs) and GTPase-activating proteins (GAPs). This is where the DrrA/Sidm effector protein plays its role. Due to its high affinity for GDP-bound Rab1, DrrA/Sidm acts as a GEF, exposing its master molecular switch allowing for the recruitment of vesicles [33]. Furthermore, previous studies have suggested that the N-terminal region of DrrA is involved in AMPylation reaction that is essential for the localization and maintaining of Rab1 in the LCV by avoiding Rab1 deactivation by GAFs [34]. These reactions are reversed through SiD and Lem3 effector proteins respectively. Further modification of Rab1 is accomplished by SidE, SdeA, SdeB, and SdeC effector proteins through a complex ubiquitination process.

L. pneumophila avoids host cell death to allow for replication by upregulation BCL-2 and blocking the activity of BNIP3 and BCL-Rambo. The only implicated factor in inhibition of BNIP3 and BCL-Rambo in past research studies had been only SidF. A recent study suggests that there is still unexplored territory pertaining to avoidance of host cell apoptosis. Speir et al. showed with mutant strains of legionella lacking SidF, that there was not any significant increase in the rate of cell death, suggesting presence of other effector proteins [35].

Past studies have shown that the LCV exploits the hosts lipid metabolism to generate a vacuole with Golgi apparatus characteristics to facilitate the hijacking of vesicles trafficked between the ER and the Golgi apparatus. The LCV acquires a composition like that of the Golgi apparatus by enriching the LCV with PtdIns4p a phosphoinositide through the T4BSS and SidF, LepB, AR1f, LecE, LpdA effector proteins. SidF in conjunction with host 5-phosphatase OCRL1 reduces PtdINs(3,4) P2 into PtdIns4P, while LpdA synthesizes phosphatic acid and LecE activates this phosphatidic acid to produce diacylglycerol, which lead to the recruitment of host Kinase D proteins with consequent recruitment of PI4IIIKB and production of PtdIns4P [35].

4. Diagnosis

4.1 Urine antigen "the rapid test"

Urinary antigen test can be used to detect Legionella. This method requires monoclonal antibodies that recognize lipopolysaccharide antigens from *Legionella pneumophila* serogroup 1 in a urine sample. Results can be available in the next few minutes, giving it an advantage for rapid diagnosis. Sensitivity ranges from 69 to 100%, and specificity ranges from 99 to 100%. One main disadvantage from this test is that it overlooks the detection from other serogroups and species of Legionella. This can be related that about 8% of patients infected with Legionella fail to excrete urine antigens [36–38].

4.2 Microbiological culture "the gold standard"

Isolation by culture continues as the gold standard for Legionella disease. It is superior to identify all of the known species and serotypes of Legionella. Sensitivity can get up to 81% and specificity range from 99%. A variety of samples from the lower respiratory tract can be used for culturing, the most commonly use is sputum. Although in these patients the disease is developed as an atypical infection, the majority of them produce little or no sputum at all. Other acceptable specimens used are fluid from bronchial aspiration, bronchial alveolar lavage, and pleural fluid. The less used are lung tissue taken from a biopsy. The most successful and selective isolation media used for Legionella is the buffered charcoal yeast extract agar, also known as BYCE agar. A positive growth is available within 3–5 days, although when it co-exists background flora, will require addition treatment to reduce it, this can delay result up to 2 weeks [39].

Environmental isolation can be also obtained by culture test but requires a various preparation techniques to decrease the presence of environmental flora from samples, as well as different media. [37, 40]

4.3 Direct fluorescent antibody "the confirmatory technique"

The using of this test helps to confirm a suspected overgrowth of Legionella in a culture. After 3 days of incubation, a direct fluorescent antibody applies to the specimen staining the viability to growth. Sensitivity for L. pneumophila serogroup-1 ranges up to 70% and specificity is 99%. Quick results can be possible to obtain, but requires expert techniques [41–43].

5. Treatment

For *Legionella pneumophila*, a high-level of suspicion and prompt initiation of adequate antimicrobial therapy is critical to improve clinical outcomes. Failure to administer proper antimicrobial therapies at an early stage of the infection has been associated with higher mortality rates [44]. The correct choice of antibiotic depends not only in its in vitro bactericidal or bacteriostatic activity, but also in its ability to penetrate the cell membrane of host tissue. This is because Legionella resides within host tissue cells. The preferred families of antibiotic are the fluoroquinolones (levofloxacin and moxifloxacin) and the macrolides (azithromycin) [45, 46].

The situations suggesting pneumonia by Legionella are: Gram stains of respiratory samples revealing many polymorphonuclear leukocytes with few or no organisms, hyponatremia, pneumonia with prominent extrapulmonary manifestations (diarrhea, confusion, etc.), failure to respond to administration of beta-lactams, aminoglycoside antibiotics, or both and recent traveling [46–48]. When treating *Legionella pneumophila*, the first choice of antibiotics should be macrolides or quinolones. Quinolones are more active than macrolides. Sometimes may be preferred in other patients whom drug interactions could be a problem. For example, in immunocompromised patients the potential for interaction with medications like cyclosporine or protease inhibitors is documented to be in a less with quinolones than with macrolides.

Azithromycin is the drug of choice for children with suspected or confirmed Legionella disease. Erythromycin is not often used now even though it is highly effective, but its use has been related with considerable side effects (i.e., gastrointestinal and ototoxicity), especially when used intravenously. Azithromycin has been shown to be the more active macrolide against *Legionella pneumophila* followed in order of activity by erythromycin, roxithromycin, dirithromycin, and clarithromycin [44, 47, 49]. Azithromycin is the safest macrolide. The advantage is due to its good intracellular penetration, bactericidal activity, proven clinical efficacy, short duration of treatment and good safety profile. Furthermore, the

15-membered lactone ring of Azithromycin does not interact with cytochrome P450 (CYP) 3A4 isoenzymes (i.e., cyclosporine). Unlike the other types of macrolides, this reduces the potential for drug interactions. The initial course should be intravenously administered. After a good clinical response is detected, it can be switched to the oral route. In patients with severe disease or unresponsive to monotherapy, the addition of rifampin is recommended [45, 50]. The recommended Azithromycin dose is 500 mg IV/PO q24h for 5 days. Alternatives are: Clarithromycin 500 mg IV/PO q12h for 10 days and Erythromycin 1 g IV q6h or 500 mg PO q6h [47].

Quinolones have all been shown to inhibit the intracellular growth of *L. pneumophila*. The most potent inhibitors of intracellular multiplication, in order of decreasing activity, were levofloxacin, ciprofloxacin, and ofloxacin [45]. Levofloxacin stops multiplication of bacteria by preventing the reproduction and repair of their genetic material (DNA) and it appears to be associated with a more rapid resolution of symptoms, a shorter time to clinical stability and consequently shorter length of hospital stay then the macrolides. Levofloxacin, either 500 mg PO/IV qd for 10 days or 750 mg PO/IV qd for 5 days, can cure most of the patients and is becoming the antibiotic of choice for Legionella disease [45, 49, 51].

Other alternatives include Doxycycline 100 mg PO/IV q12-24h for 7–21 days or sulfamethoxazole/trimethoprim DS 800 mg/160 mg 1–2 tabs PO q12h or 20 mg/kg/day IV q6-12h for 7–10 days [47, 49]. Rifampicin is very active against extracellular and intracellular Legionella spp. In the clinical setting, monotherapy is not recommended. In case Rifampicin resistance emerges, it has been reserved for adjunctive therapy in severe cases of Legionella infection. Another limitation of Rifampicin is the potent induction of cytochrome P450 enzyme system and the potential for drug interactions [45].

The usual duration of therapy for most antibiotics is 5–10 days. This is often adequate to completely treat patients with Legionella infection. Although, a duration of therapy up to 3 weeks may be considered in immunocompromised patients or in patients with severe disease or with other pre-existing health conditions (chronic heart, lung, liver or renal disease, diabetes mellitus, alcoholism, malignancies, and asplenia) [44]. Patients should be switched from intravenous to oral therapy when they are hemodynamically stable and present a clinical improvement and, also, if they are able to ingest medications and have a normally functioning gastrointestinal tract. Before discontinuation of therapy the patients should be afebrile for 48–72 hours and should be have at least one criteria for clinical stability (Temperature $\leq$ 37.80°C, heart rate $\leq$ 100 beats/minutes, respiratory rate $\leq$ 24 breaths/minutes, systolic blood pressure $\geq$ 90 mm Hg, arterial oxygen saturation $\geq$ 90% or $pO_2 \geq 60$ mm Hg on room air, normal mental status and ability to maintain oral intake). Patients should be discharged home as soon as they are clinically stable, and they have no other medical problem. Additionally it is important to have a safe environment for continuity of care. The inpatient observation while receiving oral therapy is not required [44, 51, 52].

6. Prevention

Even though *Legionella pneumophila* is a very uncommon etiology of nosocomial infection, the CDC recommends a high degree of suspicion when there are cases of nosocomial pneumonia with unknown etiology [53]. The presence of warm water is suitable for the growth of the bacteria (20–45°C). It is known that Legionella colonizes hot water distribution systems in 12–70% of hospitals in some geographic areas. For example, a study made in Hungary showed that Legionella was found in 90% of some surveyed hospitals that were >30 years old [54]. Also, it is documented that Legionella can survive at higher temperatures (>60°C) but keeping a hot water at that range can cause third-degree burns in some patients (1 second of exposure to hot water in children, and 5 seconds of exposure to hot water in adults). It is important that hospital regulations focus on maintaining proper water temperatures [55].

The frequent monitoring of hospital water system is mandatory when there is Legionella pneumonia documented in a patient hospitalized, or even when there is suspicion of Legionella. Water sample cultures are the most prevalent method for ascertaining colonization of water. The interpretation of Legionella testing can vary from geographical area, but some facilities can act and start the management of Legionella contamination when the culture results show a level of detection of 1 CFU/mL [56].

A water management program is indispensable for Legionella prevention, and it should be implemented in every hospital since the incidence has been rising up in the United States. A survey developed in Minnesota in 2017, was applied in 137 acute-care, critical care, and long-term hospitals. Only 84 surveys were returned and 3 were incomplete and excluded from the analyses. From them, 27% of the hospitals had a pertinent water management program. The 7% of those facilities measured pH at which cold and hot water were stored. The temperature range of the hot water storage was reported to be 42–62°C. All of the hospitals were supplied by community drinking water sources. Less than 5 used secondary disinfection systems (i.e., reverse osmosis, ultraviolet light, or chlorine). Also, only 21% of the responding facilities have reported to regularly test the water for the presence of Legionella [57]. They concluded that significant water management should be put into practice to protect patients from nosocomial Legionella [58].

In some other countries like Italy and Australia have developed programs for control and preventive measure for legionellosis. In Northern Italy, the water systems are routinely tested for Legionella. A questionnaire was applied to 739 hospitals, and 178 were completed. It showed that 97% of the hospitals do routine tests for the presence of Legionella in water, and 62% detected a positive result. The most common control measure is disinfection of water systems, mostly with thermal shock and chlorine dioxide [59]. Also, the implementation of a water safety plan and disinfection with monochloramine prevented legionellosis in another hospital in Catania, Italy. The results after 3 years of application have proven to be highly effective in controlling the growth of Legionella and thus preventing nosocomial infections [60].

In Brisbane, Australia, they use genomic epidemiological methods to execute a rapid and effective water treatment to characterize and eradicate *L. pneumophila*. This was started to be used due to a background of two proven nosocomial cases of *L. pneumonia*. The trace of the whole genome sequence analysis was initiated from isolates of affected patients and a prospective isolated were collected from hospital water distribution systems. The aggressive intervention to resolve this included the closure of the hospital, scalding of the water system with 60°C for 10 minutes, and treatment with alkaline detergent and 10 mg/L free chlorine, as well as the installation of in-line chlorinator systems and intensive monitoring for the presence of LPSG1 in water specimens. The combinations of all these approaches proved to be a good support in the management of Legionella contamination [61].

7. Conclusions

Legionnaires' disease is a potential preventable disease. The access to clean water should be essential for all the hospital environments, though, *Legionella pneumophila* is quite atypical. The implementation of certain methods like avoiding critical spots and the prevention of water stagnation will help to decrease the risk of proliferation of the gram-negative bacteria, as well as its growth and spreading throughout the healthcare facilities. Most hospital water systems are complex and different one from another, and this is a reason for maintenance of an adequate temperature, such as >60°C water temperature is recommended. Though, the prevention of damage to patients (third-degree burns) should be taken in consideration. This could be an alternative for prevention of the bacterial dissemination. The recalling in the pathophysiology of the bacteria will help us understand the natural history of the disease and thus comprehend our best choice for diagnosis and treatment. The diagnosis of patients with *Legionella pneumophila* is also quite important, and the microbiological culture should be used as a gold standard. The treatment needs to be initiated as soon as Legionella is suspected, and the patients should be placed in isolated rooms. Failure to starting the treatment will increase the risk of mortality among the patients. Further studies should be done to evaluate strategies of prevention of dissemination of the disease in all healthcare facilities, including the successful approaches that have been already performed in some other countries.

Conflict of interest

The authors have nothing to disclose.

Notes/Thanks/Other declarations

We want to thank Dr. Salim Surani for inviting us to participate in this book chapter.

Author details

Yamely Mendez[1*], Gloria Rueda[2], Ismael Garcia[1] and Johanan Luna[3]

1 Faculty of Medicine "Dr. Alberto Romo Caballero", Autonomous University of Tamaulipas, Houston, TX, USA

2 Health Faculty, Surcolombiana University, Houston, TX, USA

3 Faculty of Medicine, Xochicalco University, Mexicali, BC, Mexico

*Address all correspondence to: mhym2010@gmail.com

References

[1] Dooling KL, Toews KA, Hicks LA, et al. Active bacterial core surveillance for legionellosis—United States, 2011-2013. Morbidity and Mortality Weekly Report. 2015;**64**:1190-1193

[2] World Health Organization. Legionella and the Prevention of Legionellosis. Geneva, Switzerland: World Health Organization; 2007. Available from: http://www.who.int/water_sanitation_hea lth/emerging/legionella.pdf

[3] Van Kenhove E, Dinne K, Janssens A, Laverge J. Overview and comparison of Legionella regulations worldwide. American Journal of Infection Control 2019;**00**:1-11

[4] Cloutman-Green E, Barbosa VL, Jimenez D, Wong D, Dunn H, Needham B, et al. Controlling *Legionella pneumophila* in water systems at reduced hot water temperatures with copper and silver ionization. American Journal of Infection Control. 2018;**00**:1-6

[5] Borella P, Bargellini A, Marchegiano P. Hospital-acquired Legionella infections: An update on the procedures for controlling environmental contamination. Annali di Igiene. 2016;**2**:98-108

[6] Springston JP, Yocavitch L. Existence and control of Legionella bacteria in building water systems: A review. Journal of Occupational and Environmental Hygiene. 2017;**2**:124-134

[7] Herwaldt LA, Marra AR. Legionella: A reemerging pathogen. Current Opinion in Infectious Diseases. 2018;**31**:1-9

[8] Decker BK, Harris PL, Toy DL, Muder RR, Sonel AF, Clancy CJ. Water cultures are more sensitive than swab cultures for the detection of environmental Legionella. Infection Control and Hospital Epidemiology. 2018;**39**(1):108-110

[9] GLIMP Study Group, Gramegna A, Sotgiu G, Di Pasquale M, Radovanovic D, Terraneo S, et al. Atypical pathogens in hospitalized patients with community-acquired pneumonia: A worldwide perspective. BMC Infectious Diseases. 2018;**18**(1):677. (pp. 1-11)

[10] Leiblein TW, Tucker M, Ashall M, Lee SB, Gollnisch C, Hofer S. Legionella and risk management in hospitals—A bibliographic research methodology for people responsible for built environment and facility management. International Journal of Hygiene and Environmental Health. 2016;**219**(8):890-897

[11] Soda EA, Barskey AE, Shah PP, Schrag S, Whitney CG, Arduino MJ, et al. Vital signs: Health care-associated legionnaires' disease surveillance data from 20 states and a large metropolitan area—United States, 2015. American Journal of Transplantation. 2017;**17**(8):2215-2220

[12] Centers for Disease Control and Prevention. Legionella (Legionnaires' disease and Pontiac fever). Available from: https://www.cdc.gov/legionella/surv-reporting.html [Accessed: 26 October 2018]

[13] Domingo-Pueyo A, Sanz-Valero J, Wanden-Berghe C. Legionelosis ocupacional en mayores de 18 años: revisión sistemática. Ciência & Saúde Coletiva. 2019;**24**(3):793-804

[14] De Filippis P, Mozzetti C, Messina A, D'Alò GL. Prevalence of Legionella in retirement homes and group homes water distribution systems. Science of the Total Environment. 2018;**643**:715-724

[15] MacIntyre CR, Dyda A, Bui CM, Chughtai AA. Rolling epidemic of Legionnaires' disease outbreaks in small geographic areas. Emerging Microbes and Infections. 2018;**7**(1):1-10

[16] Marchesi I, Cencetti S, Marchegiano P, Frezza G, Borella P, Bargellini A. Control of Legionella contamination in a hospital water distribution system by monochloramine. American Journal of Infection Control. 2012;**40**(3): 279-281

[17] Casini B, Baggiani A, Totaro M, Mansi A, Costa AL, Aquino F, et al. Detection of viable but non-culturable legionella in hospital water network following monochloramine disinfection. The Journal of Hospital Infection. 2018;**98**(1):46-52

[18] Vincenti S, de Waure C, Raponi M, Teleman AA, Boninti F, Bruno S, et al. Environmental surveillance of Legionella spp. colonization in the water system of a large academic hospital: Analysis of the four-year results on the effectiveness of the chlorine dioxide disinfection method. Science of the Total Environment. 2019;**657**:248-253

[19] Oliva G, Sahr T, Buchrieser C. The life cycle of *L. pneumophila*: Cellular differentiation is linked to virulence and metabolism. Frontiers in Cellular and Infection Microbiology. 2018;**8**(3):1-12

[20] Eisenreich W, Heuner K. The life stage-specific pathometabolism of *Legionella pneumophila*. FEBS Letters. 2016;**590**(21):3868-3886

[21] Jäger J, Marwitz S, Tiefenau J, Rasch J, Shevchuk O, Kugler C, et al. Human lung tissue explants reveal novel interactions during *Legionella pneumophila* infections. Infection and Immunity. 2014;**82**(1):275-285

[22] Misch EA. Legionella: Virulence factors and host response. Current Opinion in Infectious Diseases. 2016;**29**(3):280-286

[23] Cazalet C, Rusniok C, Brüggemann H, Zidane N, Magnier A, Ma L, et al. Evidence in the legionella pneumophila genome for exploitation of host cell functions and high genome plasticity. Nature Genetics. Nov 2004;**36**(11):1165-1173

[24] O'Connor TJ, Zheng H, VanRheenen SM, Ghosh S, Cianciotto NP, Isberg RR. Iron limitation triggers early egress by the intracellular bacterial pathogen *Legionella pneumophila*. Infection and Immunity. 2016;**84**(8):2185-2197

[25] Mendis N, McBride P, Saoud J, Mani T, Faucher SP. The LetA/S two-component system regulates transcriptomic changes that are essential for the culturability of *Legionella pneumophila* in water. Scientific Reports. 2018;**8**(1):6764

[26] Molofsky AB, Swanson MS. *Legionella pneumophila* CsrA is a pivotal repressor of transmission traits and activator of replication. Molecular Microbiology. 2003;**2**:445-461

[27] Xu L, Luo Z-Q. Cell biology of infection by *Legionella pneumophila*. Microbes and Infection. 2013;**15**(2):157-167

[28] Meir A, Chetrit D, Liu L, Roy CR, Waksman G. Legionella DotM structure reveals a role in effector recruiting to the type 4B secretion system. Nature Communications. 2018;**9**(1):507

[29] Oot RA, Couoh-Cardel S, Sharma S, Stam NJ, Wilkens S. Breaking up and making up: The secret life of the vacuolar H^+-ATPase. Protein Science. 2017;**26**(5):896-909

[30] Zhao J, Beyrakhova K, Liu Y, Alvarez CP, Bueler SA, Xu L, et al. Molecular basis for the binding and modulation of V-ATPase by a bacterial effector protein. PLoS Pathogens. 2017;**13**(6):e1006394

[31] Yang X-Z, Li X-X, Zhang Y-J, Rodriguez-Rodriguez L, Xiang M-Q,

Wang H-Y, et al. Rab1 in cell signaling, cancer and other diseases. Oncogene. 2016;**35**(44):5699-5704

[32] Spanò S, Galán JE. Taking control: Hijacking of Rab GTPases by intracellular bacterial pathogens. Small GTPases. 2018;**9**(1-2):182-191

[33] Hardiman CA, Roy CR, AMPylation I. Critical for Rab1 localization to vacuoles containing *Legionella pneumophila*. MBio. 2014;**5**(1):e01035-e01013

[34] Qiu J, Luo Z-Q. Legionella and Coxiella effectors: Strength in diversity and activity. Nature Reviews. Microbiology. 2017;**15**(10):591-605

[35] Speir M, Vogrin A, Seidi A, Abraham G, Hunot S, Han Q, et al. *Legionella pneumophila* strain 130b evades macrophage cell death independent of the effector SidF in the absence of flagellin. Frontiers in Cellular and Infection Microbiology. 2017;7:35

[36] Avni T, Bieber A, Green H, Steinmetz T, Leibovici L, Paul M. Diagnostic accuracy of PCR alone and compared to urinary antigen testing for detection of *Legionella* spp.: A systematic review. Journal of Clinical Microbiology. 2016;**54**(2):401-411

[37] Pierre DM, Baron J, Yu VL, Stout JE. Diagnostic testing for legionnaires' disease. Annals of Clinical Microbiology and Antimicrobials. 2017;**16**(1):59

[38] Ueda A, Oki M, Yanagi H, Ozawa H, Takagi A. Clinical characteristics of *Legionella pneumonia* diagnosed with Legionella urinary antigen test. The Tokai Journal of Experimental and Clinical Medicine. 2016;**41**(1):8-13

[39] Chen DJ, Procop GW, Vogel S, Yen-Lieberman B, Richter SS. Utility of PCR, culture, and antigen detection methods for diagnosis of legionellosis. Onderdonk AB, editor. Journal of Clinical Microbiology. 2015;**53**(11):3474-3477

[40] Mercante JW, Winchell JM. Current and emerging *Legionella* diagnostics for laboratory and outbreak investigations. Clinical Microbiology Reviews. 2015;**28**(1):95-133

[41] D'Angelo A, De Simone C, Pagnottella M, Rossi S, Pepe R, Ruggieri G, et al. A case of *Legionella pneumophila* evaluated with CT and ultrasound. Journal of Ultrasound. 2017;**20**(3):243-245

[42] Herrera M, Aguilar YA, Rueda ZV, Muskus C, Vélez LA. Comparison of serological methods with PCR-based methods for the diagnosis of community-acquired pneumonia caused by atypical bacteria. Journal of Negative Results in Biomedicine. 2016;**15**(1):3. (page 1-11)

[43] Miyashita N, Horita N, Higa F, Aoki Y, Kikuchi T, Seki M, et al. Validation of a diagnostic score model for the prediction of *Legionella pneumophila* pneumonia. Journal of Infection and Chemotherapy. 2019;**25**(6):407-412

[44] Mandell L, Wunderink RG, Anzueto A, et al. Infectious diseases society of America thoracic society consensus guidelines on the management of community-acquired Pneumonia in adults. Clinical Infectious Diseases. 2007;**44**(2):S27-S72

[45] Dedicoat M, Venkatesan P. The treatment of legionnaires' disease. The Journal of Antimicrobial Chemotherapy. 1999;**43**(6):747-752

[46] Niederman MS, Mandell LA, Anzueto A. Guidelines for the management of adults with community-acquired pneumonia: Diagnosis, assessment of severity, antimicrobial therapy and prevention. American Journal of Respiratory and Critical Care Medicine. 2001;**163**:1730-1754

[47] Lokesh S, Losier A, De la Cruz C, Marion CR. Pneumonia updates on *Legionella*, *Chlamydophila* and *Mycoplasma pneumonia*. Clinics in Chest Medicine. 2017;**38**:45-58

[48] Higa F, Kusano N, Tateyama M, Shinzato T, Araki N, Kawakami K. Simplified quantitative assay system for measuring activities of drugs against intracellular *Legionella pneumophila*. Journal of Clinical Microbiology. 1998;**36**:1392-1398

[49] Cunha BA, Burillo A, Bouza E. Legionnaires' disease. Lancet. 2016;**387**(10016):376-385

[50] Garcia-Vidal C, Sanchez-Rodriguez I, Simonetti AF, et al. Levofloxacin versus azithromycin for treating *Legionella pneumonia*: A propensity score analysis. Clinical Microbiology and Infection. 2017;**23**:653-658

[51] Suchyta MR, Dean NC, Narus S, Hadlock CJ. Effects of a practice guideline for community-acquired pneumonia in an outpatient setting. The American Journal of Medicine. 2001;**110**:306-309

[52] Benenson R, Magalski A, Cavanaugh S, Williams E. Effects of a pneumonia clinical pathway on time to antibiotic treatment, length of stay and mortality. Academic Emergency Medicine. 1999;**6**:1243-1280

[53] CDC. Guidelines for preventing health-care-associated pneumonia, 2003: Recommendations of CDC and the healthcare infection control practices advisory committee (HICPAC). Morbidity and Mortality Weekly Report. 2004;**53**(RR03):1-36

[54] Barna Z, Kádár M, Kálmán E, et al. Legionella prevalence and risk of legionellosis in Hungarian hospitals. Acta Microbiologica et Immunologica Hungarica. 2015;**62**:477-499

[55] American Burn Association. Prevention scald injury educator's guide. Available from: http://ameriburn.org/wp-content/uploads/2017/04/scaldinjuryeducatorsguide.pdf [Accessed: 10 June 2019]

[56] Agarwal S, Abell V, File TM. Nosocomial (health care–associated) Legionnaire's disease. Infectious Disease Clinics of North America. 2017;**31**(1):155-165

[57] Danila RN, Koranteng N, Como-Sabetti KJ, Robinson TJ, Laine ES. Hospital water management programs for Legionella prevention, Minnesota, 2017. Infection Control and Hospital Epidemiology. 2018;**39**(3):336-338

[58] Soda EA, Barskey AE, Shah PP, et al. Vital signs: Health care associated legionnaires' disease surveillance data from 20 states and a large metropolitan area—United States, 2015. Morbidity and Mortality Weekly Report. 2015;**66**:584-589

[59] Montagna MT, De Giglio O, Napoli C, Diella G, Rutigliano S, Agodi A, et al. Control and prevention measures for legionellosis in hospitals: A cross-sectional survey in Italy. Environmental Research. 2018;**166**:55-60

[60] Coniglio M, Ferrante M, Yassin M. Preventing healthcare-associated legionellosis: Results after 3 years of continuous disinfection of hot water with monochloramine and an effective water safety plan. International Journal of Environmental Research and Public Health. 2018;**15**(8):1594. (pp. 1-11)

[61] Bartley PB, Ben Zakour NL, Stanton-Cook M, Muguli R, Prado L, Garnys V, et al. Hospital-wide eradication of a nosocomial *Legionella pneumophila* serogroup 1 outbreak. Clinical Infectious Diseases. 2016;**62**(3):273-279

Section 3

Diagnosis

Chapter 3

Legionella Pneumonia Due to Non-*Legionella pneumophila* Serogroup 1

Akihiro Ito and Tadashi Ishida

Abstract

Legionella pneumophila is one of the important pathogens in community-acquired (CAP) and hospital-acquired pneumonia that can cause severe pneumonia. Early diagnosis and treatment of *Legionella* pneumonia (LP) are essential because inappropriate therapy for *Legionella* pneumonia has been reported to worsen the prognosis. The most frequently identified causative pathogen of *Legionella* pneumonia is *Legionella pneumophila* serogroup 1. *Legionella* pneumonia due to non-*Legionella pneumophila* serogroup 1 is seen in 20% of cases. In diagnosing *Legionella* pneumonia caused by non-*Legionella pneumophila* serogroup 1, the urinary antigen test is usually negative; therefore, we need to suspect *Legionella* pneumonia by clinical information such as symptoms, vital signs, laboratory findings, and radiological findings. Based on our previous report, *Legionella* pneumonia due to non-*Legionella pneumophila* serogroup 1 was a mild to severe pneumonia. In addition, in about half of the patients, we could not suspect *Legionella* pneumonia using a six-point scoring system, which is one of the diagnostic scoring systems. Recently, a new urinary antigen test kit that could theoretically diagnose *Legionella* pneumonia due to non-*Legionella pneumophila* serogroup 1 was released in Japan. This can help in early diagnosis of *Legionella* pneumonia, including the one caused by non-*Legionella pneumophila* serogroup 1.

Keywords: diagnosis, *Legionella* pneumonia, *Legionella pneumophila* serogroup 1, non-*Legionella pneumophila* serogroup 1, urinary antigen

1. Introduction

Legionella pneumonia (LP) is caused by *Legionella* species that are important causative pathogens of community-acquired pneumonia (CAP) and hospital-acquired pneumonia. There are 58 species and three subspecies in the *Legionella* genus [1]. *Legionella* species are small to filamentous, Gram-negative rods [2].

The most frequently identified causative microorganism of *Legionella* pneumonia is *Legionella pneumophila* serogroup 1, accounting for about 80% of cases [3, 4]. In CAP, the rate of LP is reported to be 0.6–8% [5–8], although the rate differs in different areas and countries. However, in severe CAP that satisfies the Infectious Diseases Society of America/American Thoracic Society severe pneumonia criteria [9], LP is one of the most important etiologies, because the rate of LP was reported to be 13.5% in 133 patients [10] and 14.1% in 71 patients

<60 years old [11]. In addition, inappropriate initial therapy for LP was shown to be one of the independent factors predicting a worse prognosis [12]. Therefore, early and appropriate diagnosis of LP is very important to improve the prognosis of LP patients.

The gold standard in the diagnosis of LP is the identification of *Legionella* species in respiratory specimens such as sputum and bronchoalveolar lavage fluid. However, some LP patients have no sputum for culture, a dedicated culture medium, such as Wadowsky-Yee-Okuda-α or Buffered Charcoal Yeast Extract-α medium is needed, therefore identification of *Legionella* species is sometimes difficult, costly and time-consuming.

Currently, a urinary antigen test that detects soluble antigens is widely used for diagnosing LP in daily clinical practice worldwide. This diagnostic method is very useful because the examination procedure is simple and the results are known quickly. In a systematic review and meta-analysis, Shimada et al. reported that the specificity of the *Legionella* urinary antigen test was 99.1% and sensitivity was 74%; therefore, LP cannot be ruled out if this test is negative. Specifically, the sensitivity of the urinary antigen test for diagnosing LP due to non-*L. pneumophila* serogroup 1 is low [13]. Therefore, the *Legionella* urinary antigen test is not useful for diagnosing LP caused by non-*L. pneumophila* serogroup 1.

The diagnostic key for LP due to non-*L. pneumophila* serogroup 1 is to suspect *Legionella* pneumonia based on clinical information such as patients' symptoms, vital signs, laboratory findings, and radiological findings. Therefore, in this chapter, we describe the clinical characteristics of LP due to non-*L. pneumophila* serogroup 1 referred to in previous reports.

2. *Legionella* pneumonia due to non-*Legionella pneumophila* serogroup 1

2.1 Previous reports

In earlier studies, LP due to non-*L. pneumophila* serogroup 1 could be a mild to moderate pneumonia [14, 15], not only a severe pneumonia admitted to intensive care unit [16–20]. Indeed, we reported a case of LP due to *L. pneumophila* serogroup 9 in which initial treatment with single-dose oral azithromycin appeared useful, although oral levofloxacin was administered subsequently [15].

There have been many case reports of LP caused by non-*L. pneumophila* serogroup 1, but there have been few case series. Therefore, we investigated the clinical characteristics of LP due to non-*L. pneumophila* serogroup 1 and compared with LP due to *L. pneumophila* serogroup 1 [21]. There were 11 patients with LP due to non-*L. pneumophila* serogroup 1 between March 2001 and June 2016 in our hospital. Their age range was 58–82 years, and eight patients (72.7%) were male. The most common comorbidities were diabetes mellitus, chronic liver disease, and malignant disease in each of the two patients. The most common symptom was fever (72.7%), followed by cough (54.5%), and sputum (54.5%). The distribution of bacterial strains was *L. pneumophila* serogroup 3 in six patients, *L. pneumophila* serogroup 9 in three patients, *L. pneumophila* serogroup 6 in one patient, and *L. longbeachae* in one patient. As to the severity of pneumonia, about half of the cases (5/11) were mild to moderate according to the pneumonia severity index (PSI) [22], whereas most cases (10/11) were mild to moderate based on CURB-65 [23]. Five patients whose PSI class was less than IV are all improved with oral azithromycin or oral levofloxacin. In contrast, four patients were admitted to the intensive care unit, and all four patients were administered appropriate empiric antimicrobial agents, but three patients died.

2.2 Diagnostic scoring system

We cannot rule out LP by a negative result of the urinary antigen test because the sensitivity of this test is not very good. To diagnose LP with a negative urinary antigen test, we need to suspect it based on the symptoms, vital signs, laboratory examinations, and radiological findings.

In 1998, Cunha advocated a diagnostic scoring system for LP called the "Winthrop-University Hospital (WUH) criteria" [24]. The WUH criteria comprised 15 clinical findings and seven laboratory findings, and it was therefore thought to be too complicated to use in the daily clinical practice.

In 2009, Fiumefreddo proposed a six-point scoring system for predicting LP [25], and this scoring system was validated by Haubitz [26]. This scoring system comprised one symptom, one vital sign, and four laboratory findings. The criteria for the six items are listed in **Table 1**. A score ≥5 had very high specificity (99.0%) and a high positive predictive value (17.4%), whereas a score <2 had high sensitivity (94.4%) and a high negative predictive value (99.6%). In our previous reports [21], using a cutoff value of ≥2 points, the sensitivity of this scoring system was 54.5% for non-*L. pneumophila* serogroup 1 patients and 95.7% for *L. pneumophila* serogroup 1 patients. Therefore, we could not rule out LP due to non-*L. pneumophila* serogroup 1 using this six-point scoring system. In **Figure 1**, the patient number

Temperature	>39.4°C
C-reactive protein	>187 mg/L
Lactate dehydrogenase	>225 mmol/L
Platelets	<171 × 10^9/L
Serum sodium	<133 mmol/L
Unproductive cough	

Table 1.
Criteria for each item in the six-point scoring system.

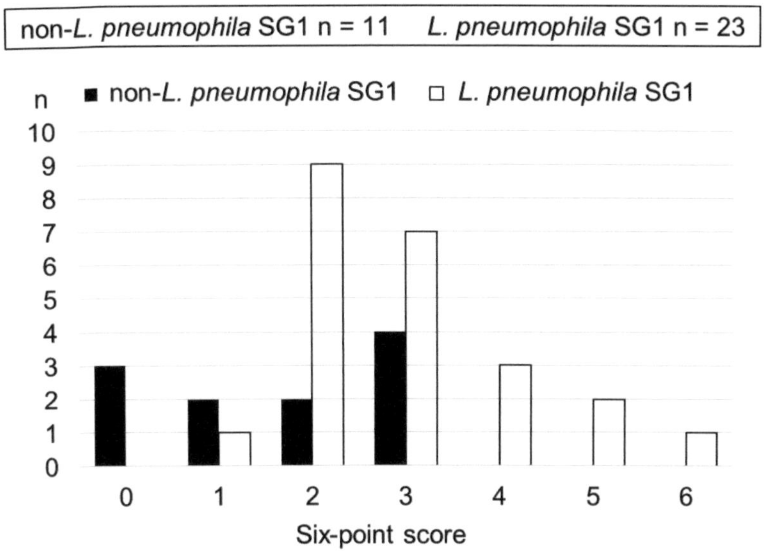

Figure 1.
Total scores of the six-point scoring system in Legionella pneumonia due to non-L. pneumophila serogroup 1 and L. pneumophila serogroup 1.

and total scores of the six-point scoring system in LP due to non-*L. pneumophila* serogroup 1 and *L. pneumophila* serogroup 1 are shown [21].

3. Future perspective

Patients with LP have a worse prognosis if they are not treated with appropriate antibiotic therapy as soon as possible. Some patients with LP due to *L. pneumophila* serogroup 1 have a negative urinary antigen test, and patients with LP due to non-*L. pneumophila* serogroup 1 are usually negative on this test. Therefore, it is important to suspect LP based on the clinical findings. However, as shown in our previous report, there are some LP patients in whom we cannot suspect LP based on the clinical findings specific to LP due to non-*L. pneumophila* serogroup 1. Thus, a simple method and a rapid test kit for diagnosing LP due to non-*L. pneumophila* serogroup 1 are needed.

In February 2019, Asahi Kasei Pharma Corporation released a urinary antigen test kit that could diagnose LP due to non-*L. pneumophila* serogroup 1, not only due to *L. pneumophila* serogroup 1. This kit uses an immunochromatographic method that has a monoclonal antibody recognizing a ribosomal protein L7/L12 unique region of *L. pneumophila* serogroups 1–15.

In the future, we expect that early diagnosis of LP including non-*L. pneumophila* serogroup 1 will be possible using this test kit.

4. Conclusion

LP due to non-*L. pneumophila* serogroup 1 can be a mild to severe pneumonia. To diagnose LP, there are some patients with LP caused by non-*L. pneumophila* serogroup 1 that could not be suspected to have LP based on their clinical findings, although diagnostic scoring systems have been reported to be useful for predicting LP. We need to investigate the usefulness of the new urinary antigen test kit that could theoretically diagnose these patients.

Acknowledgements

The authors would like to thank all of our colleagues who recruited and treated the patients. They would also like to thank Hiroyuki Fujii from the Department of Clinical Laboratory, Ohara Healthcare Foundation, Kurashiki Central Hospital, for performing sputum culture for *Legionella* species identification; Dr. Hiroshi Nakajima from the Department of Bacteriology, Okayama Prefectural Institute for Environmental Science and Public Health; and Dr. Junko Amemura-Maekawa from the Department of Bacteriology I, National Institute of Infectious Diseases, for performing *Legionella* species identification.

Conflict of interest

The authors declare no conflict of interest.

DOI: http://dx.doi.org/10.5772/intechopen.88187

Author details

Akihiro Ito* and Tadashi Ishida
Department of Respiratory Medicine, Ohara Healthcare Foundation, Kurashiki Central Hospital, Kurashiki, Okayama, Japan

*Address all correspondence to: ai12306@kchnet.or.jp

References

[1] Cunha BA, Burillo A, Bouza E. Legionnaires' disease. The Lancet. 2016;**387**:376-385

[2] Edelstein PH. *Legionella*. In: Versalovic J, Carroll KC, Funke G, Jorgensen JH, Landry ML, Warnock DW, editors. Manual of Clinical Microbiology. 10th ed. Washington, DC: American Society of Microbiology Press; 2011. pp. 770-785

[3] Amemura-Maekawa J, Kura F, Helbig JH, Chang B, Kaneko A, Watanabe Y, et al. Working Group for Legionella in Japan. Characterization of *Legionella pneumophila* isolates from patients in Japan according to serogroups, monoclonal antibody subgroups and sequence types. Journal of Medical Microbiology. 2010;**59**:653-659

[4] Helbig JH, Bernander S, Castellani Pastoris M, Etienne J, Gaia V, Lauwers S, et al. Pan-European study on culture-proven legionnaires' disease: Distribution of *Legionella pneumophila* serogroups and monoclonal subgroups. European Journal of Clinical Microbiology & Infectious Diseases. 2002;**21**:710-716

[5] Ishida T, Hashimoto T, Arita M, Ito I, Osawa M. Etiology of community-acquired pneumonia in hospitalized patients: A 3-year prospective study in Japan. Chest. 1998;**114**:1588-1593

[6] Saito A, Kohno S, Matsushima T, Watanabe A, Oizumi K, Yamaguchi K, et al. Prospective multicenter study of the causative organisms of community-acquired pneumonia in adults in Japan. Journal of Infection and Chemotherapy. 2006;**12**:63-69

[7] von Baum H, Ewig S, Marre R, Suttorp N, Gonschior S, Welte T, et al. Competence Network for Community Acquired Pneumonia Study Group. Community-acquired *Legionella* pneumonia: New insights from the German competence network for community acquired pneumonia. Clinical Infectious Diseases. 2008;**46**:1356-1364

[8] Cillóniz C, Ewig S, Polverino E, Marcos MA, Esquinas C, Gabarrús A, et al. Microbial aetiology of community-acquired pneumonia and its relation to severity. Thorax. 2011;**66**:340-346

[9] Mandell LA, Wunderink RG, Anzueto A, Bartlett JG, Campbell GD, Dean NC, et al. Infectious Diseases Society of America/American Thoracic Society consensus guidelines on the management of community-acquired pneumonia in adults. Clinical Infectious Diseases. 2007;**44**(Suppl 2):S27-S72

[10] Ishiguro T, Takayanagi N, Yamaguchi S, Yamakawa H, Nakamoto K, Takaku Y, et al. Etiology and factors contributing to the severity and mortality of community-acquired pneumonia. Internal Medicine. 2013;**52**:317-324

[11] Ishida T, Tachibana H, Ito A, Tanaka M, Tokioka F, Furuta K, et al. Clinical characteristics of severe community-acquired pneumonia among younger patients: An analysis of 18 years at a community hospital. Journal of Infection and Chemotherapy. 2014;**20**:471-476

[12] Viasus D, Di Yacovo S, Garcia-Vidal C, Verdaguer R, Manresa F, Dorca J, et al. Community-acquired *Legionella pneumophila* pneumonia: A single-center experience with 214 hospitalized sporadic cases over 15 years. Medicine (Baltimore). 2013;**92**:51-60

[13] Olsen CW, Elverdal P, Jørgensen CS, Uldum SA. Comparison of the sensitivity of the *Legionella* urinary

antigen EIA kits from Binax and Biotest with urine from patients with infections caused by less common serogroups and subgroups of *Legionella*. European Journal of Clinical Microbiology & Infectious Diseases. 2009;**28**:817-820

[14] Faris B, Faris C, Schousboe M, Heath CH. Legionellosis from *Legionella pneumophila* serogroup 13. Emerging Infectious Diseases. 2005;**11**:1405-1409

[15] Ito A, Ishida T, Tachibana H, Ito Y, Takaiwa T, Fujii H, et al. A case of community-acquired pneumonia due to *Legionella pneumophila* serogroup 9 in which initial treatment with single-dose oral azithromycin appeared useful. Japanese Journal of Infectious Diseases. 2017;**70**:660-662

[16] Chen CY, Chen KY, Hsueh PR, Yang PC. Severe community-acquired pneumonia due to *Legionella pneumophila* serogroup 6. Journal of the Formosan Medical Association. 2006;**105**:256-262

[17] Lück PC, Schneider T, Wagner J, Walther I, Reif U, Weber S, et al. Community-acquired legionnaires' disease caused by *Legionella pneumophila* serogroup 10 linked to the private home. Journal of Medical Microbiology. 2008;**57**:240-243

[18] Furugen M, Koide M, Baba M, Sato Y, Teruya H, Naha Y, et al. *Legionella* pneumonia caused by *Legionella pneumophila* serogroup 2: Second case report in Japan. Journal of Infection and Chemotherapy. 2008;**14**:161-165

[19] Kawanami T, Yatera K, Fukuda K, Yamasaki K, Kunimoto M, Nagata S, et al. Diagnosis of fulminant pneumonia caused by *Legionella pneumophila* serogroup 8 with the sequence analysis of the 16S rRNA gene. The Tohoku Journal of Experimental Medicine. 2011;**225**:65-69

[20] Grottola A, Forghieri F, Meacci M, Fabio A, Pozzi L, Marcheqiano P, et al. Severe pneumonia caused by *Legionella pneumophila* serogroup 11, Italy. Emerging Infectious Diseases. 2012;**18**:1911-1913

[21] Ito A, Ishida T, Washio Y, Yamazaki A, Tachibana H. *Legionella* pneumonia due to non-*Legionella pneumophila* serogroup 1: Usefulness of the six-point scoring system. BMC Pulmonary Medicine. 2017;**17**:211

[22] Fine MJ, Auble TE, Yealy DM, Hanusa BH, Weissfeld LA, Singer DE, et al. A prediction rule to identify low-risk patients with community-acquired pneumonia. New England Journal of Medicine. 1997;**336**:243-250

[23] Lim WS, van der Eerden MM, Laing R, Boersma WG, Karalus N, Town GI, et al. Defining community acquired pneumonia severity on presentation to hospital: An international derivation and validation study. Thorax. 2003;**58**:377-382

[24] Cunha BA. Clinical features of legionnaires' disease. Seminars in Respiratory Infections. 1998;**13**:116-127

[25] Fiumefreddo R, Zaborsky R, Haeuptle J, Christ-Crain M, Trampuz A, Steffen I, et al. Clinical predictors for *Legionella* in patients presenting with community-acquired pneumonia to the emergency department. BMC Pulmonary Medicine. 2009;**9**(4). DOI: 10.1186/1471-2466-9-4

[26] Haubitz S, Hitz F, Graedel L, Batschwaroff M, Wiemken TL, Peyrani P, et al. Ruling out *Legionella* in community-acquired pneumonia. The American Journal of Medicine. 2014;**127**:1010.e11-1010.e19

Section 4

Treatment

Chapter 4

Legionnaires' Disease Treatment

Jorge F. Velazco

Abstract

Legionnaires' disease is an important cause of community-acquired pneumonia as well as hospital-acquired pneumonia. *Legionella pneumophila* is an important but uncommon respiratory pathogen with significant morbidity and mortality. Initially recognized as a fatal cause of pneumonia in the 1970s. Untreated Legionnaires' disease conveys high mortality, therefore a prompt treatment with appropriate antibiotics is of extreme importance. Currently, therapeutic options include macrolides and fluoroquinolones mainly, that have an effective therapeutic profile. Potential issues of bacterial resistance have risen, but overall, this is not a significant limitation of therapy. In addition, attempts to identify other cases related to the case will help find potential sources.

Keywords: *Legionella pneumonia*, *Legionella pneumophila*, Legionnaires' disease, Legionellosis, antimicrobial therapy

1. Introduction

Legionella pneumophila is responsible for 90% of Legionnaires' disease (LD) [1–3]. *Legionella pneumonia*, or LD has an increasing incidence, its mortality has progressively improved from 34% in 1980, to 12% in 1998, to 3.1% in 2010, however 20–25% of patients require mechanical ventilation with a mortality rate as high as 25% [4]. It is believed that the evolution of antibiotic therapy has improved outcomes [4]. *Legionella pneumonia* may have an atypical presentation that will contribute to its underdiagnosing and under-reporting [5], majority of reported cases are due to *Legionella pneumophila* serotype-1 (80%), that may reflect the relatively wide availability of commercial kits to test for this specific serotype [5]. Legionella is an ubiquitous environmental intracellular Gram-negative bacteria, therefore antibiotics capable of penetrating phagocytic cells should be selected, then macrolides and quinolones have become the recommended therapies [6–8]. Risk factors associated with higher mortality rates are older age, smoking, chronic cardiopulmonary disease, diabetes, alcohol abuse, cancer and immunosuppression [9]. Appropriate antibiotic selection will drop mortality significantly, from 60–70% to 10–20% [2, 7, 10, 11].

2. Treatment

For years, macrolides, specifically erythromycin, has been the mainstay of therapy until the 1990s [4, 12], however with the emergence of newer macrolides and quinolones, the therapeutic selection has shifted, and now Azithromycin or Levofloxacin are considered the mainstay of LD treatment [12]. Beta-lactam and aminoglycoside antibiotics are ineffective in the treatment of LD, then empiric therapy based on either macrolides or quinolones for initial moderate to severe pneumonia will be a reasonable approach [12–14].

Effective antibiotic therapy depends on the ability to concentrate in alveolar macrophages, and for these concentrations to be effective, it will need to range from 10 to 30 times greater than serum concentrations [15] Fluoroquinolones are antimicrobials with concentration-dependent bactericidal activity [16].

In cases of severe LD, combination therapy has been advocated without evidence of superiority [12]. The incidence of LD as cause of severe pneumonia requiring ICU admission has been reported as high as second most common behind Streptococcus pneumonia (17.8 versus 21.6%, respectively) [2, 13].

In a retrospective review of 3157 adult cases, from more than 400 U.S. hospitals between 2008 and 2013, it was noted that quinolones alone were used in 28.8%, whereas azithromycin alone was used in 34% of patients, only 1.8% of patients received combination therapy (see **Figure 1**). Hence, the majority of patients with LD in the US are treated with azithromycin and/or quinolone [4]. No prospective randomized trial has compared outcomes of levofloxacin versus azithromycin [14].

2.1 Empiric therapy

The choice of empiric antibiotic therapy is based on the premise of providing optimal therapy, the epidemiological features of the probable agents, and an inference of the most likely pathogen [17].

The empirical coverage for Legionnaires' disease is still a matter of debate, in view of low testing frequency that underscores poor emphasis on Legionella role in pneumonia [18]. The incidence of LD is higher in cases of severe pneumonia, hence patients admitted to an ICU setting should be tested and treated as potential Legionella pneumonia [17]. Historically empirical optimal monotherapy treatment has been based on doxycycline, a quinolone or azithromycin [19].

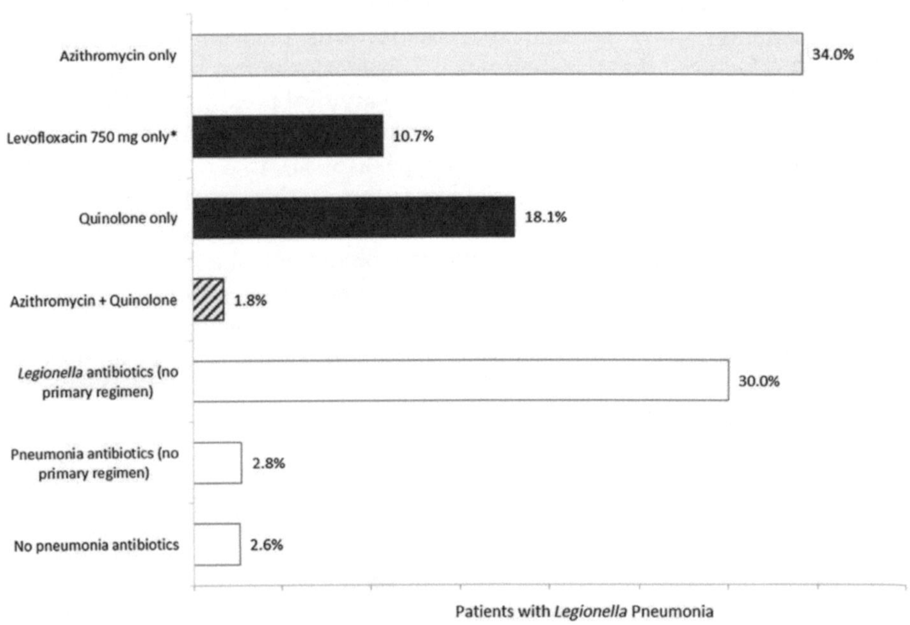

Figure 1.
In-hospital treatment strategies for patients with Legionnaires' disease. Adapted from Ref. [4].

Respiratory fluoroquinolones are an effective empiric treatment for bacterial community-acquired pneumonia, used as monotherapy in the outpatient setting, and hospitalized patients, as a first-line or alternative agents; in addition to be used as combination therapy in the ICU setting [20]. Azithromycin has a comparable antibiotic profile to fluoroquinolones, in addition has a favorable safety profile, higher intracellular concentrations and longer post antibiotic effect [21].

In a prospective observational study of 3934 hospitalized patients by Viasus et al., performed in Spain at a tertiary teaching hospital between 1995 and 2010, 214 (5.4%) patients were diagnosed with LD, and 24 patients (11.2% of the LD patients) received inappropriate empirical antibiotic therapy; among the other 190 patients, 111 received levofloxacin, 74 patients received macrolides, and three combination of quinolones and macrolides, 1 doxycycline and 1 clindamycin [22] (**Table 1**).

2.2 Targeted therapy

Early, targeted therapy that covers LD has shown to improve overall outcomes [19].

The most frequently identified of LD is *Legionella pneumophila* serogroup 1 in 80% of cases [23]. New diagnostic test had been added to the testing armamentarium (urinary antigen and polymerase chain reaction). Empirical therapy should be replaced by targeted therapy as soon as Legionella has been identified [17].

Garcia-Vidal et al. reported an observational cohort in Spain of all patients admitted with community acquired pneumonia from 2000 to 2014, 446 patients were diagnosed with LD; 335 patients (75.1%) received appropriate initial therapy with either quinolones, macrolides, combination with rifampin, or combination macrolide and quinolones. Primary outcome was overall 30-day in-hospital mortality. Thirty-six patients were excluded, 175 patients received levofloxacin, 177 patients received azithromycin and 58 patients received clarithromycin, without statistical significant difference for in-hospital 30-day mortality between the cohorts [24].

Once LD has been diagnosed, some experts suggest combined therapy instead of monotherapy for severe pneumonia, although there is no solid evidence support it [13]. In a retrospective observational multicenter Spanish series of 779 ICU patients admitted to the ICU with severe pneumonia, 25 patients (3.2%) were found to have LD, and prescription of monotherapy versus combination therapy was not

Mild disease ambulatory setting	Moderately severe disease	Severe disease intensive care unit setting
Doxycycline 100 mg orally q12h × 14d	Doxycycline 200 mg IV q12h × 72h, then 100 mg IV q12h × 11d	Doxycycline 200 mg IV q12h × 14d
Levofloxacin 500 mg orally q24h × 14d	Moxifloxacin 400 mg IV q24h × 14d	Levofloxacin 500 mg IV q24h × 14d
Moxifloxacin 400 mg orally q24h × 14d	Tigecycline 200 mg IV x 1dose, then 100 mg IV q24h × 14d	Moxifloxacin 400 mg IV q24h × 14d
Azithromycin 500 mg orally × 1dose, then 250 mg orally q24h × 10d		TMP-SMX 5 mg/kg IV q6h × 14d or Rifampin 300 mg orally q12h × 14d, maybe used as a second drug

Adapted from Ref. [15].

Table 1.
Empiric therapy for Legionnaires' disease.

protocolized, with ICU mortality as primary endpoint; it was found that there was no statistical significant difference of overall ICU mortality among both treatment groups; however if the severe pneumonia was associated to shock the difference became statistically significant [13].

2.3 Antibiotic selection and duration

There may be a role for a specific antibiotic choice based on severity of illness: need for intensive care unit (ICU) admission, need for invasive mechanical ventilation [4]. Dose and route of antibiotic delivery will be dictated by the severity, level of consciousness, and gastrointestinal function integrity [12]. Most of the antibiotics are available in oral presentations with excellent bioavailability (>90%), therefore transition among IV to oral regimens is seamless [19].

Despite absence of evidence, initial levofloxacin dose is recommended at 750 mg daily, and azithromycin 500 mg daily [14].

Levofloxacin use was associated with a shorter length of stay in the hospital, and shorter time to reach clinical stability [22]; moreover a small retrospective series showed no inferiority of ciprofloxacin to erythromycin in Japan [25]. In a retrospective single-center study at University of Michigan from 1999 to 2011, 41 patients with LD were analyzed after been treated with azithromycin versus fluoroquinolones, comparing clinical outcomes: all-cause mortality, length of stay in the hospital, time to clinical stability and development of complications, showing no significant differences among the two therapies [19, 21] (**Table 2**).

Duration of therapy is important to provide cure and prevent relapse [19]. The Infectious Diseases Society of America/American Thoracic Society (IDSA/ATS) recommend that patients with LD to be treated for 5–14 days, shorter courses maybe appropriate if Azithromycin is the antibiotic of choice. Treatment should not be stopped until patients are afebrile for 48–72 hours [22].

Therapy	Normal adult dose	Comments
Macrolides	Azithromycin 500 mg IV q24h or clarithromycin 500 mg IV q12h	Preferred regimen in most settings, or a fluoroquinolone
Fluoroquinolones	Levofloxacin 500 mg IV q24h or moxifloxacin 400 mg IV q24h	Generally well tolerated and effective
Rifampin	300–600 mg IV q12h	Multiple drug interactions, including warfarin, opiates, cyclosporine, antiretroviral protease inhibitors; used with a macrolide or quinolone
Doxycycline	200 mg IV × 1dose, then 100 mg IV q12h	Limited clinical experience shows activity
Combinations	Levofloxacin 500 mg IV q24h or another fluoroquinolone + azithromycin 500 mg IV q24h; consider adding rifampin to monotherapy	No clear evidence of efficacy of combination therapy compared with monotherapy; often used in severe extensive disease in high-risk patients falling monotherapy

Adapted from Ref. [19].

Table 2.
Therapeutic options for severe Legionnaires' disease.

Immunocompromised patients have a higher incidence of LD; cavitation, empyema, extrapulmonary disease may occur; and urinary antigen is less sensitive. In this population an antibiotic combination, and longer course maybe indicated (21 days) [3], and despite this this population has a higher mortality rate than matched groups [26]. An extended course up to 21 days is recommended for immunocompromised patients, severe disease, extrapulmonary manifestations, and inappropriate initial therapy [14].

Combination therapy has included different regimens: rifampin-clarithromycin; clarithromycin-ciprofloxacin-rifampin, and clarithromycin-levofloxacin-rifampin [13].

Older macrolides will interact with drugs like tacrolimus and ciclosporin through the cytochrome P-450 enzyme system, then quinolones, doxycycline or azithromycin maybe used in transplanted hosts [14].

2.4 Therapy outcome

Early initiation of appropriate antibiotics, improves outcomes, therapy with quinolones within 8 hours of ICU admission reduces mortality [5, 19].

In the Viasus' Spanish series, 41 (19.1%) patients with LD developed severe disease (ICU admission or death), independent factors were identified in this group: current/former smoker, macrolide use, initial inappropriate antibiotic therapy and high risk pneumonia severity index (PSI) class. The overall cure rate is 95% at 10–14 days after therapy [22] (**Table 3**).

In a Portuguese observational series, it was noted that patient with severe LD complicated by refractory respiratory failure were able to be supported by extra corporeal membrane oxygenation (ECMO) with high survival rates (86%); those patients had a faster clinical deterioration with very early ECMO initiation [27]. In a retrospective case review from University of Michigan between 1994 and 2006, survival rates were also noted to be high (67%) [28].

Antibiotic resistance is always a concern, it was noted that acquired resistance to macrolides, fluoroquinolones or rifampin could be easily selected in vitro; however in clinical practice, antibiotic susceptibility testing is not commonly performed [29], due to the fact that *Legionella pneumophila* serogroup 1 strains did not show any in vitro resistance towards eight antibiotics tested by Vandewalle-Capo et al.

Therapy and outcome	*L. pneumophila* pneumonia (*n* = 214)	*S. pneumonia* pneumonia (*n* = 1346)	P
Inappropriate antibiotic therapy	24 (11.2)	8 (0.6)	<0.001
In-hospital complications	74 (34.6)	460 (34.3)	0.92
ICU admission	38 (17.8)	151 (11.2)	0.007
Need for mechanical ventilation	26 (12.4)	122 (9.2)	0.14
Time to clinical stability, median (IQR), d	3.5 (2–5)	4 (2–6)	0.85
Length of hospital stay, median (IQR), d	9 (6–13)	8 (6–12)	0.14
Length of intravenous therapy, median (IQR), d	4 (2–6)	5 (3–7)	<0.001
In-hospital case-fatality rate	13 (6.1)	103 (7.8)	0.38

Adapted from Ref. [22].

Table 3.
Therapy and outcomes of patients with L. pneumophila and S. pneumoniae pneumonia.

(ciprofloxacin, moxifloxacin, levofloxacin, azithromycin, erythromycin, clarithromycin, rifampin and doxycycline) [1].

In a systematic review and meta-analysis comparing quinolones versus macrolides effectiveness against LD, non-significant difference was found, however all studied outcomes favored quinolones, like mortality, clinical cure, time to fever resolution, length of stay in the hospital. Twelve studies were included in the analysis, and the absence of significance maybe related to lack of statistical power [30].

3. Conclusion

Legionnaires' disease is a relative frequent cause of pneumonia syndromes, and it is associated to high morbidity and mortality [22], therefore a delay in starting appropriate therapy has been associated with increased mortality [17]. Consistent with current guidelines, antibiotic therapy should be based on either azithromycin or a quinolone to treat for Legionella pneumonia. Optimum therapy is not properly supported by clinical evidence, however in view of rare potential bacterial resistance to macrolides and quinolones, these antibiotic groups remain as mainstay of LD therapy.

Conflict of interest

The author declares no conflict of interest related to this topic.

Author details

Jorge F. Velazco
Department of Medicine, Texas A&M Health Science Center—College of Medicine, Baylor Scott and White Health-Memorial Hospital, Temple, Texas, USA

*Address all correspondence to: jorge.velazco@bswhealth.org

References

[1] Vandewalle-Capo M, Massip C, Descours G, et al. Minimum inhibitory concentration (MIC) distribution among wild-type strains of *Legionella pneumophila* identifies a subpopulation with reduced susceptibility to macrolides owing to efflux pump genes. International Journal of Antimicrobial Agents. 2017;**50**:684-689. DOI: 10.1016/j.ijantimicag.2017.08.001

[2] Harris NJ, Harris AC, Spiro M. Management of Legionella in the intensive care setting. BMJ Case Reports. 2011;**2011**:1-7. DOI: 10.1136/bcr.12.2010.3587

[3] Lanternier F, Ader F, Pilmis B, et al. Legionnaire's disease in compromised hosts. Infectious Disease Clinics of North America. 2017;**31**:123-135. DOI: 10.1016/j.idc.2016.10.014

[4] Gershengorn HB, Keene A, Dzierba AL, et al. The association of antibiotic treatment regimen and hospital mortality in patients hospitalized with *Legionella pneumonia*. Clinical Infectious Diseases. 2015;**60**:e66-e79. DOI: 10.1093/cid/civ157

[5] Sharma L, Losier A, Tolbert T, et al. Pneumonia updates on *Legionella*, *Chlamydophila*, and *Mycoplasma pneumonia*. Clinics in Chest Medicine. 2017;**38**(1):45-58. DOI: 10.1016/j.ccm.2016.11.011

[6] Miyashita N, Higa F, Aoki Y, et al. Clinical presentation of *Legionella pneumonia*: Evaluation of clinical scoring systems and therapeutic efficacy. Journal of Infection and Chemotherapy. 2017;**23**:727-732. DOI: 10.1016/j.jiac.2017.09.001

[7] Beaute J. Legionnaires' disease in Europe, 2011 to 2015. Euro Surveillance. 2017;**22**(27):1-8. DOI: 10.2807/1560-7917.ES.2017.22.27.30566

[8] Harrison CF, Kicka S, Trofimov V, et al. Exploring anti-bacterial compounds against intracellular *Legionella*. PLoS ONE. 2013;**8**(9):1-13. DOI: 10.1371/journal.pone.0074813

[9] Cecchini J, Tuffet S, Sonneville R, et al. Antimicrobial strategy for severe community-acquired legionnaires' disease: A multicenter retrospective observational study. The Journal of Antimicrobial Chemotherapy. 2017;**72**:1502-1509. DOI: 10.1093/jac/dkx007

[10] Kakeya H, Ehara N, Fukushima K, et al. Severe Legionnaires's disease successfully treated using a combination of fluoroquinolone, erythromycin, corticosteroid, and sivelestat. Internal Medicine. 2008;**47**:773-777. DOI: 10.2169/internalmedicine.47.0677

[11] Garcia-Vidal C, Carratala J. Current clinical management of Legionnaires' disease. Expert Review of Anti-Infective Therapy. 2006;**4**(6):995. DOI: 10.1586/14787210.4.6.995

[12] Phin N, Parry-Ford F, Harrison T, et al. Epidemiology and clinical management of Legionnaires' disease. The Lancet Infectious Diseases. 2014;**14**:1011-1021. DOI: 10.1016/S1473-3099(14)70713-3

[13] Rello J, Gattarello S, Souto J, et al. Community-acquired *Legionella pneumonia* in the intensive care unit: Impact on survival of combined antibiotic therapy. Medicina Intensiva. 2012;**37**(5):320-326. DOI: 10.1016/j.medin.2012.05.010

[14] Cunha B, Burillo A, Bouza E. Legionnaires' disease. Lancet. 2016;**387**:376-385. DOI: 10.1016/S0140-6736(15)60078-2

[15] Cunha CB, Cunha BA. Antimicrobial therapy for Legionnaires'

disease: Antibiotic stewardship implications. Infectious Disease Clinics of North America. 2017;**31**:179-191. DOI: 10.1016/j.idc.2016.10.013

[16] Obrink-Hansen K, Hardlei TF, Brock B, et al. Moxifloxacin pharmacokinetic profile and efficacy evaluation in empiric treatment of community-acquired pneumonia. Antimicrobial Agents and Chemotherapy. 2015;**59**:2398-2404. DOI: 10.1128/AAC.04659-14

[17] Diederen BM. *Legionella* spp. and Legionnaires' disease. The Journal of Infection. 2008;**56**:1-12. DOI: 10.1016/j.jinf.2007.09.010

[18] Gramegna A, Sotgiu G, Di Pasquale M, et al. Atypical pathogens in hospitalized patients with community-acquired pneumonia: A worldwide perspective. BMC Infectious Diseases. 2018;**18**:677. DOI: 10.1186/s12879-018-3565-z

[19] Chahin A, Opal SM. Severe pneumonia caused by *Legionella pneumophila*. Differential diagnosis and therapeutic considerations. Infectious Disease Clinics of North America. 2017;**31**:111-121. DOI: 10.1016/j.idc.2016.10.009

[20] Garau J, Fritsch A, Arvis P, et al. Clinical efficacy of moxifloxacin versus comparator therapies for community-acquired pneumonia caused by *Legionella* spp. Journal of Chemotherapy. 2010;**22**(4):264-266. DOI: 10.1179/joc.2010.22.4.264

[21] Nagel JL, Rarus RE, Crowley AW, et al. Retrospective analysis of azithromycin versus fluoroquinolones for the treatment of *Legionella pneumonia*. P&T: A Peer-reviewed Journal for Formulary Management. 2014;**39**(3):203-205

[22] Viasus D, Di Yacovo S, Garcia-Vidal C, et al. Community-acquired *Legionella pneumophila* pneumonia. A single-center experience with 214 hospitalized sporadic cases over 15 years. Medicine. 2013;**92**:51-60. DOI: 10.1097/MD.0b013e31827f6104

[23] Ito A, Ishida T, Tachibana H, et al. A case of community-acquired pneumonia due to *Legionella pneumophila* serogroup 9 wherein initial treatment with single-dose oral azithromycin appeared useful. Japanese Journal of Infectious Diseases. 2017;**70**:660-662. DOI: 10.7883/yoken.JJID.20176.548

[24] Garcia-Vidal C, Sanchez-Rodriguez I, Simonetti AF, et al. Clinical Microbiology and Infection. 2017;**23**:653-658. DOI: 10.1016/j.cmi.2017.02.030

[25] Haranga S, Tateyama M, Higa F, et al. Intravenous ciprofloxacin versus erythromycin in the treatment of *Legionella pneumonia*. Internal Medicine. 2006;**46**:353-357. DOI: 10.2169/internalmedicine.46.6006

[26] Pedro-Botet ML, Garci-Cruz A, Tural C, et al. Severe Legionnaires' disease successfully treated with levofloxacin and azithromycin. Journal of Chemotherapy. 2006;**18**(5):559-561. DOI: 10.1179/joc.2006.18.5.559

[27] Roncon-Albuquerque R Jr, Vilares-Morgado R, van der Heijden GT, et al. Outcome and management of refractory respiratory failure with timely extracorporeal membrane oxygenation: Single-center experience with *Legionella pneumonia*. Journal of Intensive Care Medicine. 2019;**34**(4):344-350. DOI: 10.1177./0885066617700121

[28] Bryner B, Miskulin J, Smith C, et al. Extracorporeal life support for the adult respiratory distress syndrome due to severe *Legionella pneumonia*. Perfusion. 2014;**29**(1):39-43. DOI: 10.1177/0267659113497229

[29] Wilson RE, Hill RL, Chalker VJ, et al. Antibiotic susceptibility of *Legionella pneumophila* strains isolated in England and Wales 2007-12. The Journal of Antimicrobial Chemotherapy. 2018;**73**:2757-2761. DOI: 10.1093/jac/dky253

[30] Burdet C, Lepeule R, Duval X, et al. Quinolones versus macrolides in the treatment of legionellosis: A systematic review and meta-analysis. The Journal of Antimicrobial Chemotherapy. 2014;**69**:2354-2360. DOI: 10.1093/jac/dku159

Section 5

Advances in Treatment

Chapter 5

Advances in Treatment and Outcomes of Patients with *Legionella* Infection

Gilda Diaz-Fuentes, Ravish Singhal and Sindhaghatta Venkatram

Abstract

Manifestations of *Legionella* infections range from benign, mild disease to a more severe form with increased morbidity and mortality, especially in untreated patients. Despite diagnostic advances, clinical diagnosis remains elusive. Macrolides and respiratory fluoroquinolones remain the antibiotics of choice for treatment of *Legionella*; however, several new antibiotics are currently under development or in clinical trials. The recommended duration of antibiotics is 5–7 days; although, some critically ill or immunosuppressed patients may require longer treatment. In vivo resistance to these antibiotics is rare, and there is no evidence that combination therapy is more beneficial than monotherapy. Early suspicion, diagnosis, and treatment are paramount for improving outcomes.

Keywords: *Legionella*, treatment, pneumonia, outcomes, antibiotics

1. Introduction

Initial recognition of Legionnaires' disease dates back to 1976 during an outbreak of respiratory illness in Philadelphia, PA at an American Legion convention [1]. The *Legionellaceae* family is extensive and contains more than 40 species, but less than half produce disease in humans, with *Legionella pneumophila* being the most common [2]. *Legionella* infections usually manifest in two forms. The most benign presentation is Pontiac fever, which typically presents as an acute, febrile, upper respiratory tract infection (non-pneumonic) that is often unrecognized and resolves spontaneously [3]. The most severe presentation is Legionnaires' disease, caused by *Legionella pneumophila*. It is an atypical pneumonia, generally affecting the lungs and gastrointestinal tract [4]. The disease affects people of all ages and causes significant morbidity and mortality, especially in patients with certain comorbid conditions. An estimated 10,000–18,000 people worldwide are infected with *Legionella* each year [5].

In a recent review, most *Legionella* pneumonia cases were reported in the Northern hemisphere. Common workplaces associated with this infection were industrial settings, office buildings, and healthcare facilities [6]. *Legionella* pneumonia was associated with mortality in 4.1% of all cases.

The clinical and radiological manifestations of *Legionella* are nonspecific. As a result, if suspected, empiric antibiotics treatment is recommended to improve

IntechOpen

morbidity and mortality associated with the disease [7, 8]. The goal of this review is to provide a concise discussion regarding indications for treatment of *Legionella*, update the information about antibiotic management, and discuss outcomes of the disease.

2. Pathogenesis

Legionella are aerobic, Gram-negative, facultative, intracellular bacilli found widely in the environment; they have been isolated from many water sources and often colonize manufactured water systems. Humans are infected by exposure to water contaminated with *Legionella*. Person-to-person transmission has been demonstrated in only one case thus far and is not considered to be a primary means of transmission. Thus, the human body may be considered a "dead-end" for *Legionella*. *Legionella* can cause sporadic and potentially life-threatening infections in immunocompromised individuals, especially the young and elderly.

Infection begins when humans inhale *Legionella*, which travels to the lower respiratory tract where the organism binds to alveolar macrophages and engulfed into the phagosomal vacuoles (also known as phagosomes). *Legionella* then blocks fusion of the phagosome with lysosomes, preventing the release of lysosomal enzymes that destroy bacterial cells. Consequently, the bacteria can freely divide in the phagosome. Eventually, the cell ruptures, releasing bacteria that can infect other cells, resulting in inflammation and sepsis. Given the lifecycle of *Legionella*, an effective antibiotic requires both anti-*Legionella* activity and a high intracellular minimum inhibitory concentration in alveolar macrophages [9]. Antibiotics that have demonstrated clinical effectiveness in Legionnaires' disease include macrolides, fluoroquinolones, tetracyclines, trimethoprim-sulfamethoxazole (TMP-SMX), and rifampin [9]. We describe the details of each of these antibiotics below.

3. Treatment

3.1 Macrolides

Bacterial ribosomes have two subunits (30S and 50S) that function in protein synthesis. In contrast, the ribosomes in animal cells have 40S and 60S subunits, and this difference ensures that different classes of antibiotics are active against bacteria and not human cells. Macrolides are bacteriostatic agents that bind reversibly to the 50S ribosomal subunit and inhibit protein synthesis [10]. They are active against a wide range of bacteria, including intracellular pathogens such as *Legionella*. Macrolides, especially azithromycin, reach peak concentration in 2–3 hours and are rapidly absorbed and distributed throughout body tissues and with good cell distribution [10]. In the past, macrolides, especially erythromycin, have been the drug of choice for treatment of Legionnaires' disease. A newer derivative, azithromycin, recently surpassed erythromycin, because azithromycin has fewer side effects and fewer interactions with other drugs than erythromycin or its counterpart, clarithromycin.

Despite macrolides' effectiveness, bacteria have developed multiple resistance mechanisms to these drugs. One mechanism is an active efflux pump to pump the drug out of the cell. Another resistance mechanism involves changing the ribosomal subunit, either by inducing genes to produce a methylase enzyme (*ermA*, *ermB*, and *ermC*) that modifies the ribosome target or by causing chromosomal mutation of the 50S ribosomal subunit. Changes in the ribosomal subunit structure decrease drug binding to the ribosome and result in decreased efficacy of the drug [10].

Common side effects of macrolides include gastrointestinal disturbances like dyspepsia, anorexia, flatulence, and arthralgias, and disturbance in taste and smell. Rarely, hepatitis, hepatic failure, thrombocytopenia, interstitial nephritis, photosensitivity, and renal failure are observed [10]. A prolonged QTc is more common with older macrolides, such as erythromycin and clarithromycin. Azithromycin, even is taken with antacids, appears to be free of drug interactions." Caution is advised, nevertheless, when using azithromycin in conjunction with drugs known to interact with erythromycin [10].

3.2 Fluoroquinolones

Along with macrolides, fluoroquinolones (levofloxacin, moxifloxacin, and ciprofloxacin) have increasingly become a drug of choice against *Legionella*. These drugs have broad-spectrum activity against Gram-positive and Gram-negative organisms, such as *Legionella* [11]. Fluoroquinolones inhibit DNA gyrase subunit A, a bacterial enzyme that relieves the tension produced when DNA unwinds during replication. Binding to DNA gyrase inhibits the transcription of bacterial DNA, resulting in bacterial cell death. Levofloxacin has an advantage in treating pneumonia, as this drug has two to five times higher concentrations in lung tissue than in serum. Bioavailability for levofloxacin is 99% for oral and intravenous (IV) medications [11]. Fluoroquinolones exhibit concentration-dependent antimicrobial activity [12].

Bacterial resistance to quinolones mostly occurs by chromosomal mutations to the DNA gyrase gene, resulting in reduced affinity of the drug to the enzyme. Also, similar to macrolides, alterations in drug efflux or cell membrane porin channels can occur, decreasing the intracellular concentration of drug [11].

Side effects of fluoroquinolones include benign rash, headaches, nausea, vomiting, diarrhea, prolonged QTc, and arrhythmia. Tendonitis and tendon rupture have been reported in young and elderly patients. Fluoroquinolones can also cause liver dysfunction. Many over-the-counter (e.g., iron, calcium, zinc, and non-steroidal anti-inflammatory drugs) and prescription medications (e.g., warfarin) can interact with levofloxacin [13].

3.3 Tetracyclines

Tetracyclines are a class of antibiotics that include doxycycline, minocycline, tetracycline, and tigecycline. These drugs are reversible competitive inhibitors and inhibit protein synthesis at the level of the ribosome via inhibition of the codon-anticodon interaction between tRNA and mRNA. These antibiotics block binding of tRNA to the 30S ribosomal subunit, thus preventing the addition of new amino acids for protein building. Because this process is reversible, these drugs are bacteriostatic [14].

Resistance to tetracyclines is acquired via bacterial conjugation, where plasmids or transposons containing resistance genes are transferred to the previously sensitive bacteria. The resistance genes produce modified bacterial porins, preventing uptake of the tetracyclines into the bacterial cell. Other mechanisms of resistance include increased drug efflux, decreased ribosomal binding, and enzymatic inactivation [14].

Tetracyclines can cause many adverse effects, including several that are life-threatening. Tetracyclines concentrate in growing teeth and bones and thus should be avoided by children and pregnant patients [14]. Additionally, tetracyclines can cause nephrotoxicity and hepatotoxicity due to fatty degeneration. Pregnant women are at increased risk of hepatotoxicity, and tetracyclines can potentiate the nephrotoxic effects of aminoglycosides and other nephrotoxic drugs. Furthermore, tetracyclines can induce photosensitivity in persons exposed to the sun during treatment [14].

3.4 Trimethoprim-sulfamethoxazole

TMP-SMX is one of the most widely used antibiotics in the world. Sulfonamides such as SMX are competitive inhibitors of para-aminobenzoic acid, and TMP inhibits dihydrofolate reductase to block the formation of tetrahydrofolate, a key cofactor in the construction of purine, thymidine, DNA, and amino acids [15]. Bacterial dihydrofolate reductase is inhibited 50–60,000 times more than mammalian enzymes; thus, this antibiotic has minimal effect on human cells [15]. Both sulfonamides and TMP act synergistically and have maximal activity when the concentration of SMX is 20 times greater than that of TMP.

Although well tolerated, TMP-SMX can cause many gastrointestinal side effects, including nausea, vomiting, and anorexia as well as rash. Sulfonamides can cause skin rashes, including hypersensitivity reactions that can progress from a mild reaction to erythema multiforme as Stevens-Johnson syndrome. Rarely, TMP-SMX can cause aplastic anemia, agranulocytosis, and fulminant hepatic necrosis [15]. Sulfonamides can cause hemolytic anemia in patients with glucose-6-phosphate dehydrogenase deficiency.

3.5 Rifampin

Rifampin is also effective against *Legionella*, as this drug inhibits bacterial and mycobacterial RNA synthesis by binding to the beta subunit of DNA-dependent RNA polymerase to prevent RNA transcription [16]. Rifampin is absorbed readily and has good penetration into the lungs and pleural fluid. Depending on concentrations reached in the infected cell and the susceptibility of the organism, rifampin can exert either bactericidal or bacteriostatic effects [16]. Most bacteria develop resistance to rifampin as the result of a gene mutation in the beta subunit of DNA-dependent RNA polymerase. Rifampin therapy is recommended only for patients with severe disease or significant comorbid conditions (e.g., poorly controlled diabetes, tobacco use, or obstructive lung disease) including immunocompromised hosts and those refractory to conventional monotherapy regimens. Significant adverse drug events and drug-drug interactions should be considered with the use of rifampin.

Rifampin should not be used as monotherapy but rather can provide a significant synergistic effect when used in combination with other antibiotics such as macrolides or quinolones [17].

Oral and IV dosing is equivalent. Rifampin induces many hepatic CYP450 isoenzymes and can enhance the metabolism of endogenous substrates, including adrenal hormones, thyroid hormones, and vitamin D. Other side effects include maculopapular rash, fever, nausea, and vomiting. Furthermore, this antibiotic can cause *Clostridium difficile* colitis, hepatitis, and liver toxicity and can result in yellow, red, or orange discoloration of bodily fluids. Soft contact lenses may be permanently stained. Rifampin can also cause postnatal hemorrhages in the mother and infant [16] (**Table 1**).

DOI: http://dx.doi.org/10.5772/intechopen.88481

3.6 Drug dosing and duration

A summary of the most common antibiotics used with doses and duration can be seen below in **Table 1**.

Antibiotic	Administration	Dose	Frequency	Duration (days)
Ciprofloxacin	IV	200–400 mg	Every 12 hours	10
		or		
	Oral	500 mg	Every 12 hours	10
Levofloxacin	IV or oral	500 mg	Daily	7–14
Moxifloxacin	IV or oral	400 mg	Daily	14
Azithromycin	IV or oral	500 mg	Daily	7–10
Erythromycin	IV	1 g	Every 6 hours	10–14
Doxycycline*	IV or oral	200 mg	Twice a day	3
	IV or oral	100 mg	Twice a day	11

**Doxycycline administered 200 mg 2×/day for 3 days followed by 100 mg 2×/day for 11 days.*

Table 1.
Recommended drug dosing and duration for antibiotics effective against Legionella.

3.7 Macrolides compared with fluoroquinolones

Previous studies have shown that patients treated with older macrolides have a higher recurrence of disease after antibiotics are withdrawn. Levofloxacin and azithromycin appear to be the ideal drugs against *Legionella* because re-growth is not observed. In fact, numerous societies, including Infectious Diseases Society of America, British Thoracic Society, and the Dutch Association of Chest Physicians, recommend fluoroquinolones or azithromycin as the preferred antimicrobial therapy for *Legionella* [18]. Comparison of levofloxacin with azithromycin in the treatment of *Legionella* has shown no difference between the two antibiotics regarding time to defervescence, time to achieve clinical stability, length of IV therapy, or length of hospital stay [12].

Other antibiotics potentially effective for *Legionella* include tigecycline. A small study in eight patients with *Legionella* suggest tigecycline as potential second-line agent for treatment of patients with severe Legionnaire's responding poorly to conventional first line agents such as levofloxacin and azithromycin [19].

4. Outcomes

A majority of patients with *Legionella* pneumonia have favorable outcomes. Mortality ranges from 1.8 to 10%. Mortality is higher in patients with sporadic infections compared to outbreak-related cases [20, 21]. Mortality is also higher in patients with hospital-acquired legionellosis, transplant recipients with unusual presentations, and missed diagnosis with negative urinary antigen [22, 23]. ICU admissions vary based on severity and underlying conditions, especially immunocompromised status.

Clinical features of *Legionella* infection in immunocompromised patients include infection (most commonly presenting as pneumonia), cavity, and empyema. Extrapulmonary disease can be present, and the urine antigen test is less sensitive [24]. There are no differences in mortality rates, length of hospital stay, development of *C. difficile* infection, or hospital costs based on chosen therapy (fluoroquinolones versus azithromycin) [25].

4.1 *Legionella* pneumonia and extracorporeal membrane oxygenation (ECMO)

Patients with *Legionella* pneumonia with severe acute respiratory distress syndrome can be treated with ECMO. Several case reports describe the outcomes of patients with *Legionella* pneumonia requiring ECMO [26–28]. With respect to outcomes for refractory respiratory failure in patients with *Legionella* pneumonia, Roncon et al. reported that 14 of 112 patients treated with ECMO had *Legionella* pneumonia [29]. *Legionella* pneumonia was associated with earlier ECMO initiation, higher static compliance and a non significant trend towards hospital survival.

4.2 HIV infection and *Legionella* pneumonia

Legionella pneumonia in HIV-infected patients is uncommon; however, some studies suggest that it occurs 40 times more frequently in patients with AIDS than in the general population [30–32]. There are also conflicting reports on the severity and outcomes of HIV infection and *Legionella* pneumonia [33]. A recent review reported that the incidence of *Legionella* pneumonia occurs in 6% of bacterial pneumonias in HIV infected patients [34]. Some reasons for a lower incidence in AIDS patients include a possible protective role of *Pneumocystis jirovecii* pneumonia (PJP) prophylaxis with TMP-SMX or the failure to isolate or diagnose *Legionella* as a coinfection. A recent study revealed that *Legionella* could be found in the bronchoalveolar fluid in AIDS patients presenting with tuberculosis and PJP [35]. This study also revealed that species-specific coinfection could occur, associating *L. pneumophila* with *M. tuberculosis* and other *Legionella* species with *P. jirovecii*.

Although most of the data on *Legionella* pneumonia in HIV patients are from case reports, a recent case-matched, case-control study reported that HIV patients presenting with community-acquired *Legionella* pneumonia have similar outcomes compared to non-HIV patients. HIV infection is not associated with higher ICU admission or increased length of hospital stay in these patients [36], and the duration of therapy is similar to non-HIV patients.

4.3 Pregnancy and *Legionella* pneumonia

The estimated prevalence of antepartum pneumonia is similar to that for the non-pregnant population at 0.78–2.7 per 1000 [37]. Although *Streptococcus pneumoniae* is the most common responsible pathogen, *Legionella* has also been reported [38, 39]. *Legionella* was implicated as a causative agent in 1.2% of pneumonias in pregnancy [40]. Treatment is similar to that of non-pregnant women. Worse outcomes have not been described, and fetal demise rarely occurs [38, 39, 41]. Factors associated with favorable outcomes include a high index of suspicion, the institution of appropriate early therapy, and presentation in the late third trimester [38].

5. Conclusions

Appropriate and timely administration of antibiotics in patients suspected with *Legionella* infection is highly recommended. Macrolides and fluoroquinolones are considered the drugs of choice for treatment. In critically ill patients or those patients not responding appropriately, combination therapy should be considered with careful evaluation of side effects and drug interactions. As for other infections, outcomes are not only related to the choice of antibiotics but also specific host factors and aggressive supportive measures. Furthermore, it is important to review antibiotic resistance patterns not only in clinical patients but also in environmental strains that are a potential source of the clinical infections [18].

Conflict of interest

The authors have no conflict of interest to declare.

Author details

Gilda Diaz-Fuentes[1,2]*, Ravish Singhal[1,2] and Sindhaghatta Venkatram[1,2]

1 Department of Medicine, Division of Pulmonary and Critical Care, BronxCare Health System, Bronx, NY, USA

2 Icahn School of Medicine at Mount Sinai, NY, USA

*Address all correspondence to: gfuentes@bronxcare.org

References

[1] Fraser DW et al. Legionnaires' disease: Description of an epidemic of pneumonia. The New England Journal of Medicine. 1977;**297**(22):1189-1197

[2] Dedicoat M, Venkatesan P. The treatment of Legionnaires' disease. The Journal of Antimicrobial Chemotherapy. 1999;**43**(6):747-752

[3] Kaufmann AF et al. Pontiac fever: Isolation of the etiologic agent (*Legionella pneumophilia*) and demonstration of its mode of transmission. American Journal of Epidemiology. 1981;**114**(3):337-347

[4] Cunha BA, Burillo A, Bouza E. Legionnaires' disease. Lancet. 2016;**387**(10016):376-385

[5] Herwaldt LA, Marra AR. Legionella: A reemerging pathogen. Current Opinion in Infectious Diseases. 2018;**31**(4):325-333

[6] Principe L, Tomao P, Visca P. Legionellosis in the occupational setting. Environmental Research. 2017;**152**:485-495

[7] Sharma L et al. Atypical pneumonia: Updates on *Legionella*, *Chlamydophila*, and *Mycoplasma* pneumonia. Clinics in Chest Medicine. 2017;**38**(1):45-58

[8] Carratala J, Garcia-Vidal C. An update on legionella. Current Opinion in Infectious Diseases. 2010;**23**(2):152-157

[9] Cunha CB, Cunha BA. Antimicrobial therapy for Legionnaire's disease: Antibiotic stewardship implications. Infectious Disease Clinics of North America. 2017;**31**(1):179-191

[10] Bakheit AH, Al-Hadiya BM, Abd-Elgalil AA. Profiles Drug Substances Excipients and Related Methodology. Vol. 39. 2014. pp. 1-40

[11] Wimer SM, Schoonover L, Garrison MW. Levofloxacin: A therapeutic review. Clinical Therapeutics. 1998;**20**(6):1049-1070

[12] Garcia-Vidal C et al. Levofloxacin versus azithromycin for treating legionella pneumonia: A propensity score analysis. Clinical Microbiology and Infection. 2017;**23**(9):653-658

[13] Ewig S, Tuschy P, Fatkenheuer G. Diagnosis and treatment of legionella pneumonia. Pneumologie. 2002;**56**(11):695-703

[14] Chopra I, Hawkey PM, Hinton M. Tetracyclines, molecular and clinical aspects. The Journal of Antimicrobial Chemotherapy. 1992;**29**(3):245-277

[15] Smilack JD. Trimethoprim-sulfamethoxazole. Mayo Clinic Proceedings. 1999;**74**(7):730-734

[16] Glatman-Freedman A. Rifampin. Pediatrics in Review. 1996;**17**(8):294-295

[17] Varner TR et al. Role of rifampin-based combination therapy for severe community-acquired *Legionella pneumophila* pneumonia. The Annals of Pharmacotherapy. 2011;**45**(7-8):967-976

[18] Sharaby Y et al. Antimicrobial agent susceptibilities of *Legionella pneumophila* MLVA-8 genotypes. Scientific Reports. 2019;**9**(1):6138

[19] Slawek D et al. Tigecycline as a second-line agent for Legionnaires' disease in severely ill patients. Open Forum Infectious Diseases. 2017;**4**(4):ofx184

[20] Dominguez A et al. Factors influencing the case-fatality rate of Legionnaires' disease. The International Journal of Tuberculosis and Lung Disease. 2009;**13**(3):407-412

[21] Sopena N et al. Sporadic and epidemic community legionellosis: Two faces of the same illness. The European Respiratory Journal. 2007;**29**(1):138-142

[22] Sivagnanam S et al. Legionnaires' disease in transplant recipients: A 15-year retrospective study in a tertiary referral center. Transplant Infectious Disease. 2017;**19**(5)

[23] Jespersen S et al. Clinical features and predictors of mortality in admitted patients with community- and hospital-acquired legionellosis: A Danish historical cohort study. BMC Infectious Diseases. 2010;**10**:124

[24] Lanternier F et al. Legionnaire's disease in compromised hosts. Infectious Disease Clinics of North America. 2017;**31**(1):123-135

[25] Gershengorn HB et al. The association of antibiotic treatment regimen and hospital mortality in patients hospitalized with *Legionella* pneumonia. Clinical Infectious Diseases. 2015;**60**(11):e66-e79

[26] Harris DJ, Duke GJ, McMillan J. Extracorporeal membrane oxygenation for legionnaires disease: A case report. Critical Care and Resuscitation. 2002;**4**(1):28-30

[27] Jones NC. Outbreak of legionnaires' disease in the United Kingdom. Extracorporeal membrane oxygenation should be considered in severe cases. BMJ. 2 Nov 2002;**325**(7371):1033

[28] Madurka I et al. Successful extracorporeal membrane oxygenation (ECMO) treatment in *Legionella* pneumonia. Orvosi Hetilap. 2019;**160**(6):235-240

[29] Roncon-Albuquerque R Jr et al. Outcome and management of refractory respiratory failure with timely extracorporeal membrane oxygenation: Single-center experience with *Legionella* pneumonia. Journal of Intensive Care Medicine. 2019;**34**(4):344-350

[30] Pedro-Botet ML et al. Legionnaires' disease and HIV infection: An opportunistic infection? Medicina Clínica (Barcelona). 2004;**123**(15):582-584

[31] Pedro-Botet ML et al. Legionnaires disease and HIV infection. Chest. 2003;**124**(2):543-547

[32] Stroup JS, Hendrickson SE, Neil M. Legionella pneumonia and HIV infection: A case report. The AIDS Reader. 2004;**14**(5):267-270

[33] Sandkovsky U et al. *Legionella* pneumonia and HIV: Case reports and review of the literature. AIDS Patient Care and STDs. 2008;**22**(6):473-481

[34] Benito N et al. Pulmonary infections in HIV-infected patients: An update in the 21st century. The European Respiratory Journal. 2012;**39**(3):730-745

[35] Head BM et al. Legionella co-infection in HIV-associated pneumonia. Diagnostic Microbiology Infectious Disease. 14 Mar 2019. pii: S0732-8893(18)30315-8

[36] Cilloniz C et al. Community-acquired *Legionella* pneumonia in human immunodeficiency virus-infected adult patients: A matched case-control study. Clinical Infectious Diseases. 2018;**67**(6):958-961

[37] Kaunitz AM et al. Causes of maternal mortality in the United States. Obstetrics and Gynecology. 1985;**65**(5):605-612

[38] Eisenberg VH et al. Legionnaire's disease during pregnancy: A case presentation and review of the literature. European Journal of Obstetrics, Gynecology, and Reproductive Biology. 1997;**72**(1):15-18

[39] Vimercati A et al. Legionnaire's disease complicating pregnancy: A case report with intrauterine fetal demise. Journal of Perinatal Medicine. 2000;**28**(2):147-150

[40] Lim WS, Macfarlane JT, Colthorpe CL. Pneumonia and pregnancy. Thorax. 2001;**56**(5):398-405

[41] Gaillac N et al. *Legionella pneumophila* pneumonia during pregnancy: A case report. The Journal of Infection. 2006;**52**(6):e163-e164

Section 6

Legionnaires' Disease in Immunocompromised Host

Chapter 6

Legionnaires Disease in Immunocompromised Host

Venkat Rajasurya and Salim Surani

Abstract

Legionella bacteria are aerobic, pleomorphic, gram negative bacilli found in fresh water environments and are usually transmitted through inhalation aerosols from contaminated water or soil. Legionnaire's disease is a severe form of pneumonia caused by legionella species and can be community acquired or hospital acquired. The reported incidence of Legionnaires' disease is approximately 1.4–1.8 cases per 100,000 persons and immunocompromised state is a very important risk factor. Some of the other important risk factors include old age, impaired cellular immunity, hematologic malignancies, solid organ transplantation, splenectomy, tumor necrosis factor-alpha inhibitors, chronic respiratory disease, diabetes and end stage renal disease. *Legionella pneumophila* serotype 1 is the most commonly reported cause of human Legionella infections. The pathogenesis of legionnaire's disease involves invasion of alveolar macrophages and cell mediated immunity is the primary means of immune control. The prevalence of Legionnaires disease has risen possibly from increased awareness and reporting. The symptoms of the disease are nonspecific requiring a high index of suspicion in vulnerable hosts, as effective treatment could be life-saving. Sensitivity of urinary antigen testing is lower in immunocompromised patients because of higher likelihood of infections caused non L. pneumophila species. Extrapulmonary manifestations and higher mortality are particularly more common in immunocompromised patients than in immunocompetent hosts.

Keywords: transplant, legionnaires' disease, immunocompromised patients, immunocompromised hosts

1. Introduction

Legionnaire's disease is a severe form of atypical pneumonia caused by gram-negative bacteria Legionella [1]. Although Legionnaire's disease is commonly reported in immunocompetent patients, immunocompromised state, particularly impaired cellular immunity is an independent risk factor for legionella infection. Diabetes, hematologic malignancies, chronic corticosteroid use, solid organ transplantation, TNF-alpha inhibitors are all risk factors for development of legionella infection [2]. *Legionella micdadei*, *Legionella longbeachae*, *Legionella bozemanae*, *Legionella dumoffii* and *Legionella feeleii* are some of the non-pneumophila species that predominantly cause infections in individuals with impaired immunity [3]. In immunosuppressed patients legionella can disseminate outside the lungs causing extrapulmonary manifestations like skin abscess, cellulitis, septic arthritis, myocarditis, endocarditis, peritonitis etc. [4]. Secondary to the increased incidence

Legionella testing should be routinely done in immunosuppressed patients presenting with symptoms suggestive of Community acquired pneumonia.

2. Anti-Legionella immunity

Legionella pneumophila is an intracellular pathogen that replicates within alveolar macrophages. There are more than 60 species of legionella and out of which, serogroup 1 causes majority of legionella disease. Humans become infected after inhaling contaminated aerosols. *L. pneumophila* then enters and replicates within the lung alveolar macrophages. Bacteria are initially engulfed by phagocytes from a vacuole that blocks phagolysosome fusion by delivering bacterial proteins into host cell cytosol [5]. These proteins subsequently modulate endoplasmic reticulum and prevent lysosomal mediated killing of the bacteria. Another defense mediator of the body involves toll like receptors (TLR) on host cells, which senses various signaling proteins produced by *L. pneumophila*. This is in turn induces transcription factor, nuclear factor kappa B and produces inflammatory cytokines that sets up a potent immune response against *L. pneumophila*. A common genetic variation of the stop codon in the ligand binding domain of TLR increases the risk of acquiring legionella infection [6].

Tumor necrosis factor alpha is vital in protecting the body from *L. pneumophila* infection and the incidence of Legionnaires disease is reported to be higher in patients receiving TNF-alpha antagonists when compared to controls [7]. Defective monocytic-macrophagic system seen in hematological conditions can lead to the development of Legionnaire's disease. T lymphocytes are essential for effective anti-legionella control but the exact role of B lymphocytes is unclear. Though some studies have highlighted the role of immunoglobulins during legionella infection an increased incidence of Legionnaire's disease has not been found in patients with humoral immune deficiency [8].

3. Splenectomized patients

Legionella infection has not been frequently reported in splenectomized patients as these patients primarily have impairment in humoral immune response and B-lymphocyte function. A case report in 2004 reported two cases of Legionnaire's disease in splenectomized patient. The first patient developed multiorgan failure and laboratory testing was positive for *Legionella hackeliae* and *Legionella longbeachae*. The second patient was positive for *Legionella micdadei* [9]. Another patient with hairy cell leukemia and splenectomy died from multiorgan failure from *L. longbeachae* infection [10]. In 2012, *Legionella pneumophila* pneumonia was been reported in a patient with Myelodysplastic syndrome and splenectomy [11].

4. Primary immunodeficiencies

Primary immunodeficiency disorder is the result of defective immune system development and the absence of functional immune system leads to severe infections. There has been only one case of legionella pneumonia reported in a patient with primary immunodeficiency disorder. It was a 35-year-old male with hyper IgE disease who presented with hemoptysis and was later diagnosed to have cavitary pneumonia due to legionella which was isolated from the BAL cultures and the patient also had a positive urinary legionella antigen [12].

5. Organ transplant patients

Although there are many species of Legionella, *L. pneumophila* is the most common one to cause pneumonia in recipients of organ transplant. Among the non-pneumophila species, *L. micdadei*, followed by *L. longbeachae*, *L. bozemanii*, *L. parisiensis* and *L. cincinnatiensis* commonly caused pneumonia in transplant recipients [3].

A Spanish group of physicians retrospectively reviewed 287 cases of Legionnaires' disease in solid organ transplant patients. They reported that 3% of the transplant recipients had contracted Legionnaires' disease. Incidence of legionnaire's disease was variable but higher in kidney, lung and heart transplant patients [13].

Extrapulmonary manifestations of *Legionella* infection were described in four solid organ transplant patients. The extrapulmonary sites were aorta, pericardium, liver and soft tissue.

A group in Seattle, Washington reviewed 15 year longitudinal data in a hospital that cares for transplant patients and reported 32 cases of Legionnaires disease over a period of 15 years and 10 of them were in solid organ transplant patients [14].

6. Biologic agents

Biologic drugs are very commonly used for treatment of number of diseases and are associated with an increased risk of serious infections by lowering the immunity. A study done in France in 2006 over a period of 1 year revealed a case series of 10 patients treated with anti-TNF alpha therapy who were diagnosed with *Legionella pneumophila* infection [15]. Another French study that looked into risk factors for legionella infection from 2004 to 2007 concluded that anti TNF alpha therapy was associated with 13-fold increased risk of developing legionella infection. There was a 15-fold higher risk associated with infliximab, 38-fold higher risk associated with adalimumab and 3-fold increase with etanercept. Patients had different degrees of presentation. 28% presented with bilateral pneumonia, 24% had ARDS, 33% were hospitalized in ICU and 1 patient died [7]. A recent review from 2004 to 2011 reported 105 cases of Legionnaire's disease in patients treated with biologic treatment [16].

7. Malignancies

Patients with hematological and solid tumors are at higher risk for developing legionnaire's disease. A study found that Legionella caused 29% of pneumonia in patients with head and neck malignancies [17]. A retrospective study over 4 years conducted in a oncology center in 1986 found 36 cases of Legionnaire's disease. 42% had hematological malignancy and 22% had lung cancer. Neutropenic patients and patients on chronic steroids had higher risk of getting legionnaire's disease [18].

Two retrospective studies were done at MD Anderson cancer hospital in Texas. First study reported 49 cases of Legionnaire's disease in cancer patients over a period of 13 years from 1991 to 2003. The majority of patients had an underlying hematologic malignancy. 37% were bone marrow transplant recipients. Lymphopenia, use of corticosteroids and chemotherapy were the most common risk factors in these patients [19]. Second retrospective study reviewed 33 consecutive cases of Legionnaire's disease between 2002 and 2014. Out of this 27 had hematologic malignancies, 23 had neutropenia, 6 had allogeneic hematopoietic stem cell transplant and all patients except 1 had lung infection [20].

Clinical presentation of LD in immunocompromised patients:

Legionnaires disease in immunocompromised patients presents with fever, cough, chills, shortness of breath. GI symptoms can also occur. The incubation period for Legionnaires' disease is usually around 2–10 days from the time of exposure to symptom onset. In immunocompromised patients in addition to consolidation legionnaire's disease can present with cavitations, diffuse bilateral infiltrates and pleural effusions. In transplant patients nodular opacities that eventually cavitate have been reported [21]. Pleural effusions have been reported in 15–50% of cases.

Pneumonia with cavitation has been reported in L pneumophila serotypes 1, 3, 4, 5, 6, and 8 as well as other Legionella species including *L. micdadei*, *L. bozemanae*, *L. dumoffii*, and *L. longbeachae* [22]. Legionella species can also cause lung abscesses and the most important risk factor for it is prolonged use of glucocorticoid therapy. Abscesses generally arise after 4 weeks of starting high dose glucocorticoid therapy. Complicated pleural effusions, empyema and lung abscesses caused by legionella are more commonly seen in patients with solid organ transplant [23].

Extrapulmonary manifestations are usually seen in immunocompromised hosts [4]. The incidence of Neurologic manifestations including meningoencephalitis, meningitis and transverse myelitis are similar to as in immunocompetent hosts. Cutaneous legionella has been reported in patients on chronic corticosteroids, solid organ transplants, stem cell transplants and hematological malignancies. They present with erythema, nodules, induration, ulcer or abscess. Most of them have concomitant lung infection [24].

Legionella can also affect the heart. *L. pneumophila* causing aortitis has been reported in heart transplant patients. Twelve cases of pericarditis were reported and most of them were in immunocompromised patients including transplant recipients, dialysis patients and cancer patients [25].

8. Conclusion

In conclusion while Legionella infection can occur in both immunocompetent and immunocompromised patients, certain risk factors in the immunocompromised are associated with an increased incidence. T cell and cell mediated immunity play a key role in body's defense against the bacteria. TNF Alpha inhibitors are associated with an increased risk of Legionnaire's disease. Extrapulmonary manifestations involving the skin, pericardium and aorta were seen more in immunocompromised, predominantly in patients on chronic corticosteroids, solid organ and stem cell transplant patients. The incidence of neurological manifestations remained the same. The signs and symptoms of Legionnaire's disease are non-specific and patients with the above high risk features, especially on TNF alpha inhibitors should be screened for Legionella infection.

Author details

Venkat Rajasurya[1] and Salim Surani[2]*

1 Novant Health, Winston-Salem, North Carolina, USA

2 Texas A&M University, Health Science Center, College of Medicine, Texas, USA

*Address all correspondence to: srsurani@hotmail.com

References

[1] Fraser DW, Tsai TR, Orenstein W, Parkin WE, Beecham HJ, Sharrar RG, et al. Legionnaires' disease: Description of an epidemic of pneumonia. The New England Journal of Medicine. 1977;**297**(22):1189-1197

[2] Marston BJ, Lipman HB, Breiman RF. Surveillance for Legionnaires' disease. Risk factors for morbidity and mortality. Archives of Internal Medicine. 1994;**154**(21):2417-2422

[3] Chow JW, Legionella YVL. A major opportunistic pathogen in transplant recipients. Seminars in Respiratory Infections. 1998;**13**(2):132-139

[4] Sivagnanam S, Pergam SA. Legionellosis in transplantation. Current Infectious Disease Reports. 2016;**18**(3):9

[5] Roy CR, Tilney LG. The road less traveled: Transport of Legionella to the endoplasmic reticulum. The Journal of Cell Biology. 2002;**158**(3):415-419

[6] Kawai T, Akira S. The role of pattern-recognition receptors in innate immunity: Update on toll-like receptors. Nature Immunology. 2010;**11**(5):373-384

[7] Lanternier F, Tubach F, Ravaud P, Salmon D, Dellamonica P, Bretagne S, et al. Incidence and risk factors of *Legionella pneumophila* pneumonia during anti-tumor necrosis factor therapy: A prospective French study. Chest. 2013;**144**(3):990-998

[8] Schlossberg D, Bonoan J. Legionella and immunosuppression. Seminars in Respiratory Infections. 1998;**13**(2):128-131

[9] Gorelik O, Lazarovich Z, Boldur I, Almoznino-Sarafian D, Alon I, Modai D, et al. Legionella in two splenectomized patients. Coincidence or causal relationship? Infection. 2004;**32**(3):179-181

[10] Lang R, Wiler Z, Manor J, Kazak R, Boldur I. *Legionella longbeachae* pneumonia in a patient splenectomized for hairy-cell leukemia. Infection. 1990;**18**(1):31-32

[11] Cunha BA, Hage JE. *Legionella pneumophila* community-acquired pneumonia (CAP) in a post-splenectomy patient with myelodysplastic syndrome (MDS). Heart & Lung. 2012;**41**(5):525-527

[12] Di Stefano F, Verna N, Di Gioacchino M. Cavitary Legionella pneumonia in a patient with immunodeficiency due to hyper-IgE syndrome. The Journal of Infection. 2007;**54**(3):e121-e123

[13] Gudiol C, Garcia-Vidal C, Fernandez-Sabe N, Verdaguer R, Llado L, Roca J, et al. Clinical features and outcomes of Legionnaires' disease in solid organ transplant recipients. Transplant Infectious Disease. 2009;**11**(1):78-82

[14] Sivagnanam S, Podczervinski S, Butler-Wu SM, Hawkins V, Stednick Z, Helbert LA, et al. Legionnaires' disease in transplant recipients: A 15-year retrospective study in a tertiary referral center. Transplant Infectious Disease. 2017;**19**(5). DOI: 10.1111/tid.12745

[15] Tubach F, Ravaud P, Salmon-Ceron D, Petitpain N, Brocq O, Grados F, et al. Emergence of *Legionella pneumophila* pneumonia in patients receiving tumor necrosis factor-alpha antagonists. Clinical Infectious Diseases. 2006;**43**(10):e95-e100

[16] Viasus D, Di Yacovo S, Garcia-Vidal C, Verdaguer R, Manresa F, Dorca J, et al.

Community-acquired *Legionella pneumophila* pneumonia: A single-center experience with 214 hospitalized sporadic cases over 15 years. Medicine (Baltimore). 2013;**92**(1):51-60

[17] Johnson JT, Yu VL, Wagner RL, Best MG. Nosocomial *Legionella pneumonia* in a population of head and neck cancer patients. The Laryngoscope. 1985;**95**(12):1468-1471

[18] Nunnink JC, Gallagher JG, Yates JW. Legionnaires' disease in patients with cancer. Medical and Pediatric Oncology. 1986;**14**(2):81-85

[19] Jacobson KL, Miceli MH, Tarrand JJ, Kontoyiannis DP. Legionella pneumonia in cancer patients. Medicine (Baltimore). 2008;**87**(3):152-159

[20] Han XY, Ihegword A, Evans SE, Zhang J, Li L, Cao H, et al. Microbiological and clinical studies of Legionellosis in 33 patients with cancer. Journal of Clinical Microbiology. 2015;**53**(7):2180-2187

[21] Ernst A, Gordon FD, Hayek J, Silvestri RC, Koziel H. Lung abcess complicating *Legionella micdadei* pneumonia in an adult liver transplant recipient: Case report and review. Transplantation. 1998;**65**(1):130-134

[22] Ampel NM, Wing EJ. Legionella infection in transplant patients. Seminars in Respiratory Infections. 1990;**5**(1):30-37

[23] Guy SD, Worth LJ, Thursky KA, Francis PA, Slavin MA. *Legionella pneumophila* lung abscess associated with immune suppression. Internal Medicine Journal. 2011;**41**(10):715-721

[24] Padrnos LJ, Blair JE, Kusne S, DiCaudo DJ, Mikhael JR. Cutaneous legionellosis: Case report and review of the medical literature. Transplant Infectious Disease. 2014;**16**(2):307-314

[25] Scerpella EG, Whimbey EE, Champlin RE, Bodey GP. Pericarditis associated with Legionnaires' disease in a bone marrow transplant recipient. Clinical Infectious Diseases. 1994;**19**(6):1168-1170